Natural
Pregnancy

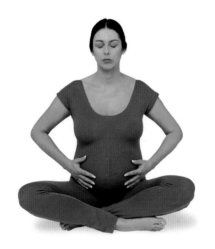

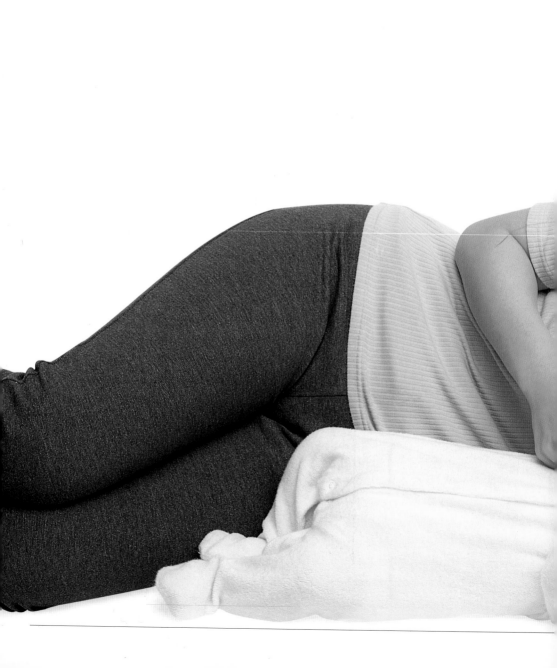

Natural Pregnancy

Zita West

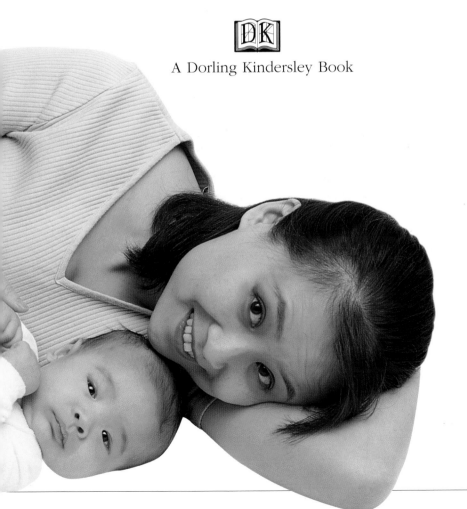

A Dorling Kindersley Book

Dorling **DK** Kindersley

London, New York, Munich,
Melbourne, Delhi

Senior Editor Jude Garlick
Senior Art Editor Dawn Terrey
Managing Editor Susannah Marriott
Managing Art Editor Clare Shedden
DTP Designer Conrad van Dyk
Production Controller Maryann Webster
Photographer Andy Crawford

You are strongly advised to consult
a conventional medical practitioner before using
any complementary treatments if you have
symptoms of illness, any diagnosed ailment
or if you are receiving conventional treatment or
medication. Do not cease conventional treatment
or medication without first consulting your
doctor. Always inform your doctor and your
complementary practitioner of any treatments,
medication or remedies that you are
taking or intend to take.

First published in Great Britain in 2001,
by Dorling Kindersley Limited
80 Strand, London WC2R 0RL
A Penguin Company

Copyright © 2001 Dorling Kindersley Limited
Text copyright © 2001 Zita West

A CIP catalogue record for this book is
available from the British Library.

ISBN 0 7513 2757 3

Reproduced by Colourscan
Printed and bound by Printer Trento Srl, Italy

See our complete catalogue at
www.dk.com

Contents

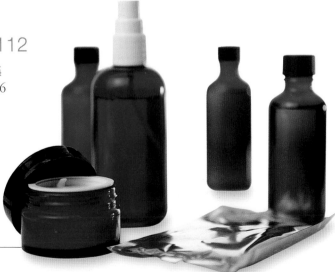

Foreword

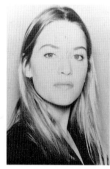

As soon as I found out that I was pregnant, I seemed to be assailed with well-meaning but conflicting advice from every direction. "You should try this", "You shouldn't do that", "You ought to eat this", "You mustn't touch that". All very confusing.

That's why this book became my bible during pregnancy. It really does contain everything you need to know, from information on diet and exercise to tips on how to deal with minor ailments and ways to prepare for labour. Most refreshing of all is that Zita doesn't preach or try to persuade you down a completely "natural" route. She "knows her stuff" but her view is a balanced one which bridges the gap between alternative and orthodox, complementary and conventional.

And she doesn't blind you with science, either. The information is comprehensive, helpful, easy to find and in short digestible chunks (and that's important when you're pregnant!). Reading the book gave me confidence and I'm sure it helped me to cope better during both pregnancy and labour.

Of all the information and advice in the book, I think what I found most fascinating was the section on docosahexaenoic acid (DHA) and how important it is for the baby's developing brain. I rushed straight out to get my own supply. I'm also certain that without Zita's dietary advice and the vitamin supplements I took, I would never have survived filming at 18 weeks.

Before I was pregnant, I thought I knew exactly how I would feel - confident, blooming and sexy – the way celebrities are expected to feel. Not a bit of it! Pregnancy turned out to be one of the hardest things I've ever done, physically, mentally and emotionally. Instead of shining hair and glowing cheeks, the reality was morning sickness, swollen ankles and a bad back, and by the third trimester I felt more like a large red London bus than a film star. Zita's suggestions for alternative remedies made all the difference. The one tip she didn't give was how to cope with hot weather - oh, the joy of sitting in a paddling pool in the garden at 34 weeks, eating ice-cream and wearing the one pair of knickers that still fit!

Kate Winslet

Introduction

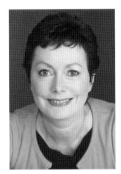

I work as a midwife and acupuncturist, both in private practice and within the UK's National Health Service. Over the years, I have treated thousands of pregnant women and observed first-hand the growing interest in holistic natural remedies and complementary therapies. During pregnancy, more than at any other time in their lives, women seek natural products, non-invasive treatments and drug-free methods of pain relief that will not harm their babies. So much rests on the healthy, happy outcome of a pregnancy that women want to be involved in their antenatal care. They are unwilling to be passive and "patient". Complementary approaches to antenatal care give a woman choice and help her to regain a feeling of control over her body. Treatments work in harmony with natural rhythms, recognizng the body's innate ability to heal itself. They focus on the person rather than the complaint.

Pregnancy is, after all, a natural physiological event, not an illness. Information, advice and support are what most women are looking for – not diagnosis or cure. Many pregnancy ailments are hard to alleviate conventionally, so orthodox medicine tends to regard them as par for the course. Most mothers-to-be would rather suffer themselves than pop a pill that might have unexpected side effects. But no woman needs to suffer pain or discomfort during pregnancy. Most minor ailments can be relieved by using a combination of complementary therapies. There is a wealth of natural remedies and treatments available – for specific conditions and to enhance general well-being – to ensure that women can enjoy their pregnancies in a state of blooming health.

I hope that this book will provide the reader with useful information – about preconceptual care, development and care in each trimester, preparation for labour, the birth, postnatal care and recommended complementary therapies. With knowledge, practical advice and sensible notes of caution will come the confidence to enjoy your pregnancy and the birth of your baby in good health and with a positive state of mind.

Zita West.

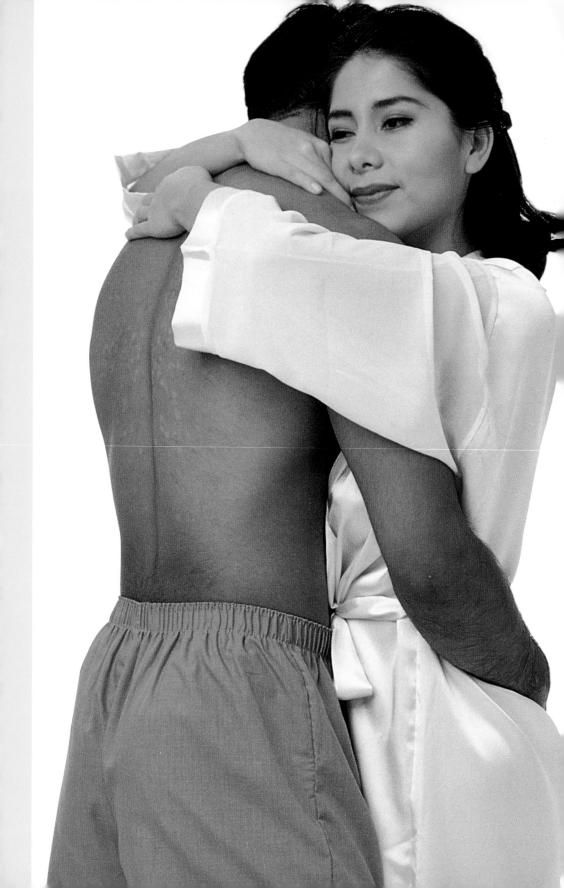

MOST PROSPECTIVE PARENTS these days are unwilling to leave having their babies to chance. More and more couples make plans for conception, pregnancy and birth in advance. Ideally, you and your partner should start to prepare four months before you want to conceive. You should both prepare yourselves physically, nutritionally,

Planning for conception & pregnancy

emotionally and mentally. This section advises you how to improve fertility and fitness prior to conception, and outlines fundamental issues relevant throughout your pregnancy. These include good nutrition, fitness, dealing with illness, your environment, and practicalities that need to be considered, such as antenatal tests.

Getting Fit for Pregnancy

HEALTHY BABIES COME FROM HEALTHY PARENTS. You and your partner should both prepare for pregnancy. Not only will this maximize your chances of conception and ensure normal, healthy sperm and eggs, it will help to protect the foetus from the risk of abnormalities during the first crucial few weeks after conception.

IMPROVING FERTILITY

Most couples take about six months to conceive, though longer is not unusual. Studies indicate that women have infertility problems in two-thirds of couples who cannot conceive and men in one-third. The health of both partners is very important. Healthy sperm and eggs (ova) are needed to reduce the risk of foetal abnormalities that may lead to miscarriage. Women who smoke are more likely to be infertile, to take longer to conceive, to miscarry and to bleed during pregnancy. If both partners smoke, there is a greater risk of the baby having a low birth weight. Women who drink and smoke are four times more likely to miscarry. Alcohol damages sperm, affects fertility and increases the risk of miscarriage and birth defects. Its effects are greatest in early pregnancy when cell division is at its peak. It is advisable not to drink alcohol from before you hope to conceive until after the birth. If you discover that you are pregnant having not stopped smoking nor reduced your alcohol consumption, do so as soon as possible. Tea and coffee deplete the body of water and valuable minerals, and they are best avoided or strictly limited, along with other drinks containing caffeine.

AVOIDING POLLUTION

Protect yourself from environmental pollution by following these guidelines whenever possible.

• Eat organic, natural and unprocessed foods; wash all fruit.
• Avoid using copper and aluminium cookware.
• Drink filtered or bottled water, not from the tap.
• Avoid heavy traffic and close car windows in tunnels.
• Avoid chemical cleaning agents and pesticides.
• Spend plenty of time outdoors, where sunlight helps to eliminate toxic substances and metabolize benefical minerals.

VITAL NUTRIENTS FOR WOMEN & MEN

NUTRIENT	WOMEN	MEN	DEFICIENCIES
VITAMIN A	*Egg production and reproductive health*	*Healthy sperm*	*Colds, infections, poor skin and hair condition*
B VITAMINS	*Prevents neural tube defects in foetus*	*Male hormone production*	*Irritability, aches and pains, anxiety*
VITAMIN C	*Builds up immunity, body detoxification*	*Improves sperm count and quality*	*Colds, infections, lack of energy*
Zinc	*Egg production and reproductive health*	*Improves sperm count and quality*	*Poor skin condition, poor taste and smell*
OTHER MINERALS	*Reproductive health (magnesium), body detoxification (selenium), balances blood sugar levels (chromium)*	*Improving sperm count (magnesium) and motility (potassium), fertility (selenium)*	*Muscle weakness (magnesium), mental dullness (potassium), nutritional disorders (selenium)*
AMINO ACIDS	*Building and repairing cells and tissues*	*Sperm health and sperm count*	*Muscle weakness, poor wound healing*

EFFECTS OF TOXIC METALS

Each year every person in the industrialized world consumes about 5 kg (11 lb) of additives, absorbs 1 g of heavy metals and has at least 4.5 litres (1 gal) of pesticides or herbicides sprayed on their fruit and vegetables. This toxic overload affects both health and fertility.

• High levels of lead can damage sperm and eggs and affect sperm count and motility. Lead accumulates if calcium, zinc, manganese and iron levels are low. Vitamin C helps to remove lead from the body.

• Mercury from pesticides and fungicides, industrial processes and dental fillings causes loss of libido and impotence.

• Aluminium, for example from saucepans, antiperspirants, food additives and foil-wrapped foods, causes longterm mineral loss and destroys vitamins.

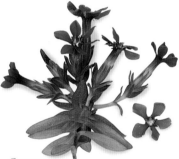

GENTIAN
This flower remedy may help to lift despondency that arises from a difficulty in conceiving.

COMPLEMENTARY THERAPIES

A number of remedies may improve health and fertility.

• Acupuncture (*see pages 134–5*) can help to regulate the menstrual cycle and correct imbalances in body systems. The Chinese believe that a person's every movement, thought, metabolic reaction and sensation is affected by *qi* (life energy), with which we are endowed from our parents at the moment of conception.

• Flower remedies may also be helpful (*see page 154*). Alpine lily encourages a positive attitude to conception and pregnancy, while bleeding heart may help relieve the grief associated with a previous miscarriage that might prevent conception. Tiger lily may help older women to conceive.

• Osteopathy and chiropractic (*see pages 146–7*) can help to realign the body and restore balance and harmony throughout so that all body parts function as they should.

• Shiatsu and reiki (*see pages 138–9*) are believed to improve the flow of *ki*, preparing body, mind and spirit for conception and pregnancy.

• Aromatherapy and massage (*see pages 152–3*) can ease stress and relieve physical tension.

Nutrition: Overall Plan

MOTHER AND BABY HAVE DIFFERENT nutritional needs at each stage of pregnancy. Ideally, you should be in peak health before becoming pregnant, so that from the moment of conception your baby has the best chance of development. A good diet throughout pregnancy will ensure your baby's optimum progress.

KEY TIPS

Make sure your diet is balanced, especially if you are vegetarian

✳

Eat lots of small meals rather than one or two large ones

✳

Avoid highly processed foods, alcohol, tobacco and caffeine

WINDOWS OF OPPORTUNITY

Research shows that while in the womb and immediately after birth, a baby's organs undergo rapid growth spurts. They develop at specific times, in a specific sequence, and for each one there is a specific window of opportunity, vital for its future health. This developmental process is known as programming. What you eat may help to maximize these opportunities. The growth of your baby's cells, tissues and organs depends upon an adequate supply of oxygen and essential nutrients. If there are shortages of these, your baby will adapt by slowing cell growth. This slow-down will be especially marked in tissues or organs that are undergoing a critical period of growth. Your health and nutritional status, at the moment of conception and throughout the pregnancy, is of crucial importance to the health and growth of your offspring.

ENERGY REQUIREMENTS

Your body becomes more energy-efficient in pregnancy, increasing your metabolic rate. This affects your need for calories. A pregnant woman's energy requirement is about 1,940 calories a day, increasing by only 200 calories in the third trimester. Appetite is the best indicator of how much to eat. Little and often is the key: five or six small but nutrient-dense meals a day are better than one or two large ones.

RATIONALIZING WEIGHT

Excessive weight gain during pregnancy concerns many women. In general, antenatal clinics no longer weigh women at every visit, it being of limited usefulness. You can weigh yourself at home, of course, remembering to use the same scales, weigh yourself at the same time of day and wear similar clothing each time. The range of weight gain during pregnancy varies, but as a

KEY FOOD TYPES

PROTEINS
These consist of amino acids – the basic building blocks of cells. Foods include meat, fish, cheese, eggs.

CARBOHYDRATES
The main sources of energy, these are simple, such as sugar, or complex, such as starch (pasta, rice, potatoes).

FATS
These are concentrated sources of energy. Some are vital for health, such as polyunsaturated fats, while others (saturated fats) may cause health problems.

VEGETARIAN PASTA
The orange and red peppers, tomatoes and cashews in this vegetarian pasta dish provide rich sources of beta carotene and vitamins C and E.

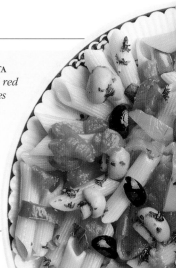

rule you can expect to gain 11–16 kg (24–35 lb): usually 3–4 kg (6–9 lb) in the first 20 weeks and then about 450 g (1 lb) a week thereafter until term. If you are underweight, your gain will be 12.5–18 kg (28–40 lb), and if you are overweight, 7–11 kg (15–25 lb).

VEGETARIAN DIET

A well-balanced vegetarian diet can be nutritionally excellent. Protein from combinations of vegetable sources, such as nuts, pulses and seeds, can be just as good as protein from meat, with the added advantage that they are full of complex carbohydrates and fibre rather than saturated fat. However, pregnant vegetarians must guard against deficiencies, particularly in vitamins B^2, B^6 and B^{12}, zinc, iron and – in the case of vegans – calcium.

MAXIMIZING ABSORPTION

It is important to understand how best to maximize the nutritional value of food.
• Eat organic food preferably and avoid processed and refined foods which contain additives and preservatives.
• Eat food when it is as fresh as possible. Cook vegetables as little as possible (but meat and eggs should be well cooked). Steam food rather than boil it and avoid frying, especially at high temperatures.
• Drink filtered rather than tap water and remember to wash all fruit and vegetables.
• Nutrients work together in synergy, so it is better to take a good multivitamin and mineral supplement than individual minerals or vitamins. Always check that they are suitable for taking during pregnancy.
• Eat a wide variety of foods and different coloured foods to include all essential nutrients. To the Chinese, a well-balanced diet means eating the five flavours of foods: sweet, sour, pungent, salty and spicy.

ANTI-NUTRIENTS

Certain substances inhibit the absorption of nutrients and therefore adversely affect nutritional status.
• The only safe level of alcohol consumption during pregnancy is no alcohol. It

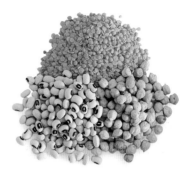

BEANS, CHICKPEAS & LENTILS
A selection of different plant sources of protein eaten every day will supply the amino acids that the body needs.

affects the body's absorption of B vitamins, calcium, iron, zinc and magnesium, and is a factor in raised blood pressure. It can cross the placenta, so if you have a drink, the baby does too.
• Smoking in pregnancy is associated with miscarriage, low birth weight and premature labour. It reduces the supply of oxygen and nutrients to the baby, reducing its growth rate and possibly damaging DNA. Nicotine increases excretion of calcium and destroys vitamin C.
• Tea and coffee have a diuretic effect and interfere with the absorption of calcium, magnesium, zinc and iron.

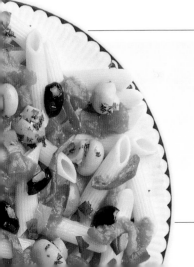

KEY NUTRIENTS NEEDED & SOURCES

CALCIUM
Milk, cheese, yogurt, pulses, nuts, tofu, wholegrains

IRON
Meat, poultry, dark oily fish, pulses, seafood, fortified grains, nuts, seeds, dried fruit, green leafy vegetables

ZINC
Meat, poultry, oysters and other shellfish, pulses, kiwi fruit

B VITAMINS (INCLUDING FOLATE)
Meat, poultry, fish, dairy products, fortified cerals, nuts, seeds, green vegetables, pulses, orange juice, bananas, avocado, wholegrains

VITAMIN C
Citrus fruits, tomatoes, red peppers, strawberries, kiwi fruit, parsley

Boosting Immunity

YOUR NATURAL IMMUNITY is slightly lowered during early pregnancy so that your body does not reject the developing baby. This is part of the normal physiological process of maintaining a pregnancy. With the increasing resistance of bacteria to antibiotics, it is important to maintain a healthy immune system.

HOW THE IMMUNE SYSTEM WORKS

Disease-producing organisms are to be found in air, food and water and on surfaces that we touch. The immune system defends the body in a number of ways. The first lines of defence are physical barriers – skin and mucous membranes. Mucus is produced by cells in the membranes and this traps bacteria or particles that have been inhaled by the respiratory tract, for example. Buying over-the-counter drugs to dry up a runny nose is not a good idea since it only prolongs this stage of the infection. If a pathogen invades the body successfully, it starts to penetrate cells and proliferate. Chemicals such as histamine in cells alert the immune system to the invader. The blood supply to that area is then increased, moving specialized white blood cells in to attack the invaders.

EFFECTS OF A WEAK SYSTEM

If your immune system is weak you are likely to suffer from recurrent coughs and colds, wounds that are slow to heal, greater fatigue than usual and bacterial, viral or fungal infections. Bacterial infections affect mucous membranes and may be accompanied by fever and swollen lymph glands. Common bacterial infections include boils and impetigo. Viruses invade cells where they replicate. Colds, influenza, warts, herpes and gastroenteritis are all viral infections. Common fungal infections include ringworm and athlete's foot.

CAUSES OF A WEAK SYSTEM

There are several factors that might inhibit or damage your natural immunity.
• Stress and anxiety depresses the immune system.
• Inadequate rest (less than eight hours' sleep a night) can debilitate the immune system.
• Food allergies exhaust the system's defences.
• Diet affects the immune system. Consuming just 80 g (3 oz) of sugar results in a 50 per cent reduction in the activity of white blood cells for between one and five hours. Poor diet generally deprives the body of the nutrients it needs

FOODS RICH IN VITAMIN C
These are good foods to eat to prevent illness from striking (see opposite).

EATING FOR HEALTH

NUTRIENT	PROTECTIVE ROLE	FOOD SOURCES
Vitamin A	*Strengthens tissues, cells and mucous membranes*	*Fish oils, egg yolks, cheese, yogurt, carrots, spinach, broccoli, tomatoes*
Vitamin C	*Fights infections, increases resistance to toxins and viruses*	*Most fruit, especially citrus and berries, potatoes, parsley*
Vitamin E	*Protects against free radicals and infections*	*Fresh nuts, seeds, cold-pressed oils*
Zinc	*Fights infections, maintains healthy immune system*	*Ginger, sunflower seeds, cold-pressed oils*
Selenium	*Enhances immune system, fights infection; anti-oxidant*	*Tuna, herring, wheatgerm, Brazil nuts, seafood, seeds*
Green foods	*Enhances immune system, protects against bacteria and viruses*	*Vegetables containing chlorophyll, the green pigment in plants*

for a healthy immune system.
• Alcohol reduces mobilization of white blood cells.
• Air pollution damages mucous membranes.
• Chronic antibiotic use causes general immune impairment.

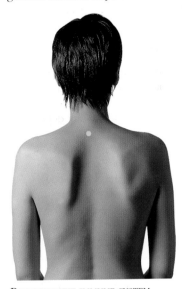

BOOSTING THE IMMUNE SYSTEM
Pressure applied to GV 14 on the back of the neck helps to increase the number of white blood cells.

USING COMPLEMENTARY THERAPIES

Good nutrition is the best foundation on which to build a healthy immune system (*see above*) There are a number of natural ways of boosting the body's immunity.
• **Acupuncture** The Chinese believe that protective *qi* surrounds the body, warding off disease. If the immune system is weak, infection may enter the body, but climatic factors such as wind, cold, heat and damp also play a role. If illness is caused by cold, then an acupuncture point may be warmed. If heat is the cause, certain acupuncture points will be used to clear heat. This therapy can be used to boost the white cell count (*see left*).
• **Aromatherapy** Tea tree oil is an effective antibacterial agent and can be applied topically to fight infection. Inhaling the vapours rising from a few drops of essential oil in hot

water may relieve respiratory infection. Anti-inflammatory oils such as chamomile, lavender, rose and sandalwood will ease bad throats or chest complaints. Breathing difficulties can be eased by using eucalyptus, mint, frankincense or tea tree oils.
• **Herbal remedies** Echinacea is a good, all-round antiviral and antibacterial herb. It can be taken continuously, as capsules or drops, throughout a period of illness, and is perfectly safe during pregnancy. Garlic contains allicin, which has antiviral, antifungal and antibacterial properties. Many regular garlic eaters have been shown to have a lower incidence of cancer. Lemon balm is good for the feverish conditions associated with viral infections, and ginger root, combined with ground cinnamon and lemon and honey to taste, makes a soothing, protective infusion for sore throats and stomach upsets.

Illness during Pregnancy

ILLNESS AND INFECTION ARE NOT KEPT AT BAY just because you have a pregnancy to maintain. The best way of preventing illness is to boost your immune system so that it can fight infection. There are safe and natural remedies that boost immunity and relieve symptoms of some common ailments that strike in pregnancy.

KEY TIPS

Fortify the immune system

✻

Avoid people with infections

✻

Rest, sleep and drink lots of fluids

✻

Consult a doctor if vomiting or diarrhoea persists

COLDS & INFLUENZA

Colds and influenza can be debilitating during pregnancy. Herbal remedies include a warming apple drink made by simmering 15 ml (1 tbsp) concentrated apple juice with 300 ml (½ pint) filtered water, 2.5 g (½ tsp) grated raw ginger, one stick cinnamon and two cloves for 15 minutes, then strain. Drink three cups a day. An infusion (*see page 150*) of elderflower, peppermint or dried yarrow may ease cold symptoms. There are many homeopathic remedies for colds.
• At the first symptoms that develop after being chilled and include a headache, *Aconite 6c*.
• Sudden onset of symptoms, fever, headache, *Belladonna 6c*.
• Aching muscles, joint pain, fever, exhaustion, *Rhus tox 6c*.
• Stuffy nose, watering eyes, headache, sore throat, better for warmth, *Nux vomica 6c*.

PARASITES

Head lice seem to be immune to medicated shampoos and have reached epidemic level among schoolchildren. If you are pregnant, avoid shampoos containing pesticides. Natural solutions include:
• Using a "nit" comb while conditioner is on the hair.
• Adding ten drops geranium or lavender oil to fractionated coconut oil (proportions half and half). Rub into the scalp and leave for one hour before washing off with shampoo.
• Applying diluted tea tree oil (with water, proportions half and half) to the scalp.

CYTOMEGALOVIRUS

Caused by a type of herpes virus, this is common during pregnancy and produces mild influenza-type symptoms. More than half of pregnant women are immune and only a small proportion of those who are not will pass the infection on to the baby, which can cause serious problems. A blood test will reveal immunity status.

CHICKEN POX

This is rare in pregnancy (one in 2,000) since most women have immunity from childhood. A blood test will reveal your immunity status. The virus is

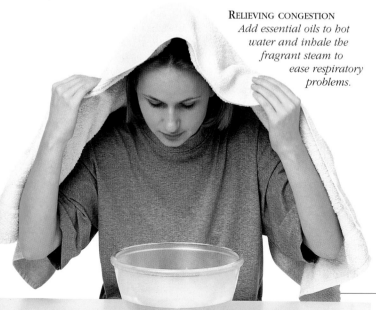

RELIEVING CONGESTION
Add essential oils to hot water and inhale the fragrant steam to ease respiratory problems.

HOMEOPATHIC REMEDIES FOR FOOD INFECTIONS

SYMPTOMS	HOMEOPATHIC REMEDY AND DOSAGE
Burning stomach pains, chilliness, anxiety, thirst, symptoms worse between midnight and 2.00 am	*Arsen. alb. 6c,* every hour for up to 10 doses
Diarrhoea, tearfulness, symptoms worse at night	*Pulsatilla 6c,* every hour for up to 10 doses
Frequent vomiting, bloating, yellow stools, chilliness, symptoms worse for eating	*China 6c,* every hour for up to 10 doses
Diarrhoea worse for movement, rumbling stomach, profuse and watery pale-coloured stools	*Phos. ac. 6c,* every hour for up to 10 doses
Burning stomach pains, blood-streaked stools, violent vomiting, craving for iced water, icy-cold extremities	*Phos. 6c,* every hour for up to 10 doses
Suspected salmonella: painless diarrhoea and fever	*Baptisia 6c,* every hour for up to 10 doses
Unremitting vomiting, foul-smelling greenish-coloured stools	*Ipecac. 6c,* every hour for up to 10 doses

spread by coughs and sneezes and is highly infectious. In the first trimester, especially weeks 1–8, it may cause birth defects, but beyond 12 weeks there is little serious risk until late pregnancy, when you should consult a doctor. Homeopathic remedies can bring relief.

• As a preventative measure if you have been in contact with chicken pox or shingles, *Rhus tox 30c* once a day for ten days.

• At onset of illness, with low fever and general discomfort, *Aconite 30c*; with fever and inflamed spots, *Belladonna 30c*.

• Unbearable itching, *Sulphur 6c*. Rub honey on to the spots, or add ten drops bergamot oil to 5 ml (1 tsp) carrier oil and dab on the spots. Five drops chamomile added to a carrier oil will soothe and heal damaged skin. Use diluted echinacea tincture (with water, half and half) to soothe itching.

FOOD INFECTIONS

Food infections are rare but it is worth avoiding certain foods in pregnancy. These include unpasteurised cheese, especially soft cheeses such as Camembert; blue veined cheeses, such as Danish blue; cook-chill foods; pâté; uncooked eggs, as in homemade ice cream and mayonnaise; and undercooked meat. Always wash fruit and vegetables thoroughly.

• Listeriosis results from eating contaminated soft cheese or chicken. The bacteria crosses the placenta. Infection in the first trimester often results in spontaneous abortion and in the second, premature labour. Infection is rare (1 in 20,000), but the bacterium can survive in temperatures as low as 4°C (39°F) – the typical temperature in a refrigerator.

• Toxoplasmosis is serious during pregnancy. Parasitic in

origin, it is contracted by eating or handling raw or undercooked meat or by touching infected cat faeces. The infection can cross the placenta and the greatest risk to the baby is from 10–24 weeks. Spontaneous abortion may occur in early pregnancy and miscarriage and still birth later on. Treatment of toxoplasmosis in pregnancy is complicated as the drugs used can also affect the foetus.

• Salmonella is a common cause of food poisoning (there are 200 different strains). It does not cross the placenta, however. There are a number of homeopathic remedies to treat food infections (*see above*). Herbal remedies include infusions of aniseed, fennel, chamomile or mint, and root ginger (a 2.5 cm /1 in length) added to hot water with a cinnamon stick, lemon juice and honey to taste.

Exercise: Overall Plan

THERE ARE MANY BENEFITS to adopting a regular exercise programme during pregnancy. Exercise will boost energy levels, maintain and promote circulation and mobility, and encourage good posture by increasing physical awareness and control. Exercise can also target certain muscles in preparation for labour.

KEY TIPS

Stop exercising if you experience serious discomfort or pain and consult your midwife or doctor

✳

Do not get overheated

✳

Limit strenuous exercise to 15 minutes' duration

PHYSIOLOGICAL CHANGES

Changes in pregnancy affect every body system and must be taken into account before exercising. Hormonal changes are highly significant. Relaxin, produced from two weeks into pregnancy and reaching a peak at 12 weeks, relaxes ligaments so that the pelvis can expand during delivery. Ligaments throughout the body are also relaxed, however, and the stability of joints is affected. It is easy to overstretch, putting the spine and pelvis at risk. Progesterone modifies the diaphragm and the ribs flare slightly to allow more room for the growing uterus. An increase in girth and weight means that your posture will change and your centre of gravity will shift. You may find it hard to co-ordinate movements and to balance. The amount of blood pumped by the heart increases by up to 40 per cent during pregnancy and the size of the heart increases to cope with this.

GENERAL GUIDELINES

Pregnancy is not the time to start aerobics classes unless they are especially structured for pregnancy. If you are used to doing such exercise and do not want to let your fitness level drop, continue but bear in mind the following guidelines.
• Your heart rate should not rise above 140 beats a minute. Do not do strenuous exercise for more than 15 minutes.

• Several research studies have indicated that intensive exercise raises the mother's core body temperature and causes vasoconstriction (the narrowing of blood vessels), which reduces blood flow and hence oxygen supply to the uterus, with a corresponding rise in the foetal heart rate.
• Increased body mass creates momentum that makes it more difficult to control movements. Jerky movements, bouncing and jumping should be avoided because impact is transmitted to the joints. Whatever stage of pregnancy you are at, be guided by your body.
• Never force yourself to exercise beyond what feels comfortable. Avoid unstable positions, such as standing on one leg for a long time. In each trimester consider the most appropriate exercise (*see pages 32–3, 50–1* and *74–5*). Always warm up before doing any exercise and cool down when you have finished (*see page 32*).

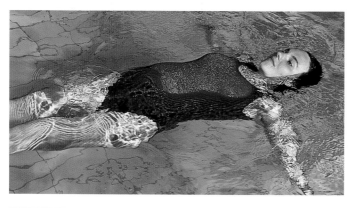

AQUAROBICS
Exercising in water is beneficial because there is less stress on the joints and on uterine blood flow.

CHOOSING EXERCISE

Seek out specially structured pregnancy fitness classes, which have a cardiovascular section, a muscle-strengthening section and a cool-down. Any strenuous exercise should be limited to 15 minutes and you should always be supervised by a teacher who is aware of the physiological changes that take place during pregnancy. Apart from exercise classes, gentle cycling is good exercise in pregnancy, although your changing centre of gravity may be a problem latterly. Walking is excellent, and speed walking is preferable to running or jogging. Swimming and water-based exercise are ideal forms of exercise. The resistance of the water enhances the effects of exercise, and strain on the back is relieved while the uterus is supported by the water. Contact sports such as hockey or netball should be avoided.

SEASONAL EXERCISE

The idea of living one's life in harmony with nature is fundamental to Traditional Chinese Medicine. In the five element theory, the seasons of the year and the changes that they bring affect our growth and well-being (*see pages 133*). The Chinese believe that exercise – as well as diet and lifestyle habits – need to be adjusted according to these seasonal changes (*see below*).

EXERCISE IN HARMONY WITH NATURE

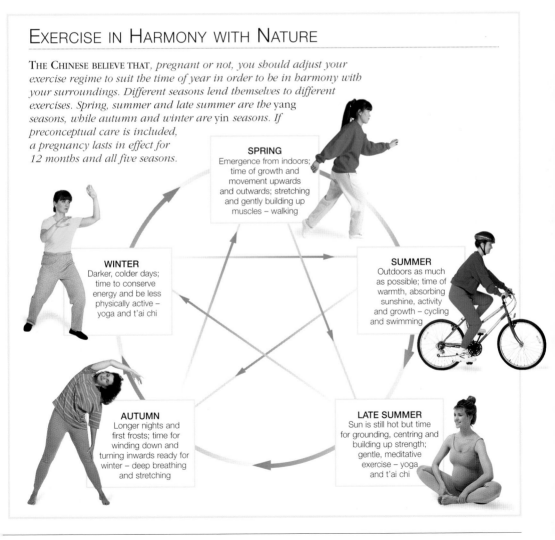

THE CHINESE BELIEVE THAT, *pregnant or not, you should adjust your exercise regime to suit the time of year in order to be in harmony with your surroundings. Different seasons lend themselves to different exercises. Spring, summer and late summer are the* yang *seasons, while autumn and winter are* yin *seasons. If preconceptual care is included, a pregnancy lasts in effect for 12 months and all five seasons.*

SPRING
Emergence from indoors; time of growth and movement upwards and outwards; stretching and gently building up muscles – walking

WINTER
Darker, colder days; time to conserve energy and be less physically active – yoga and t'ai chi

SUMMER
Outdoors as much as possible; time of warmth, absorbing sunshine, activity and growth – cycling and swimming

AUTUMN
Longer nights and first frosts; time for winding down and turning inwards ready for winter – deep breathing and stretching

LATE SUMMER
Sun is still hot but time for grounding, centring and building up strength; gentle, meditative exercise – yoga and t'ai chi

At Home & at Work

WHETHER AT HOME OR AT WORK, your surroundings exert influence over your stress levels, state of health and general well-being. Organize the places in which you spend most of your time, harnessing your natural "nesting" instincts to create harmony, positive energy and a pleasant, calm-inducing atmosphere.

KEY TIPS

Reduce stress levels

✳

Reduce exposure to pollution

✳

Make your physical surroundings pleasant and relaxing

✳

Do not "overdo it" at work

CHINESE BELIEFS

Feng shui is the Chinese art of understanding and harnessing the universal flow of *qi* energy around the home and in places of work. It is believed that this energy can be a positive force in life, for happiness, prosperity and good health. Feng shui includes a number of measures to enhance the home.

• Use mirrors and reflective surfaces to capture pleasant views from outside and reflect bad energy out of a building.

• Wind chimes and bells can help to break up stagnant *qi*, but not in a bedroom.

• Fresh flowers and plants bring good *yang* energy into a building, but always replace dead ones and avoid spiky plants and cacti. Do not put plants in a bedroom, but fruits are an excellent idea. The pomegranate, in particular, is believed to symbolize fertility.

• Air rooms and replace stale energy at least once a week by opening all the windows.

• Play loud, happy music once a week to dispel old energy and welcome in the new.

• Never hang a mirror so that it reflects a bed, which may give rise to heart problems.

• Do not sleep beneath an exposed beam. Move the bed or camouflage the beam.

• Place a bed diagonally to a door and never sleep with either your head or feet pointing directly at the door.

• A bedhead should ideally stand against a wall.

• Avoid having water features in a bedroom.

• Decorating a bedroom in red is said to stimulate passion and to bring good luck to couples wishing to start a family.

IMPROVING YOUR SURROUNDINGS
Fresh flowers, scented candles, incense, essential oils and crystals improve a room's atmosphere.

CLEARING SPACE

As you prepare to welcome a new human being into your life, find time to sort out your home and dispose of unwanted things and clutter. This will help to create space for your new baby, both literally and psychologically. If you are decorating, imagine bringing in light, happiness and harmony as you choose colours. Clear stagnant energy by a simple ceremony of clapping or sounding bells and chimes, particularly in the corners of a room. Wash your hands in running water after doing this. Then, bring in fresh flowers, light candles and incense, or spray the rooms with water containing a few drops of essential oil of lavender, mandarin or grapefruit.

AVOIDING POLLUTION

To minimalize the risks from the environment, bear in mind the following general precautions.

• Avoid standing immediately in front of a microwave oven while it is in use.

• Avoid living close to high-voltage cables during pregnancy.

• Avoid chemical hazards such as oven cleaners, garden pesticides and chemical-based cleaning agents. Check the contents of products you are using, and opt for safe, natural alternatives whenever possible.

• Avoid driving in heavy traffic and always close car windows when passing through tunnels.

• Wash all fruit and vegetables and remove the outer leaves of vegetables. Eat organic produce whenever possible.

• Avoid using aluminium or copper cookware and do not wrap food in aluminium foil.

COPING WITH WORK

Unless your work is physically demanding or the work environment is hazardous, there is no reason why you should not work through pregnancy until about 32 weeks. You may need to make some adjustments to your working day, however.

• If you spend long periods of time in front of a VDU, make sure that you sit with the screen at the correct distance and height, and that you take short, frequent breaks away from it.

• Make your day less arduous by sitting down as much as possible, putting your feet up and resting if at all possible (*see below*). Do not be afraid to ask for help if you need it and take a break if you feel fatigued.

• Make sure that you know the details of your maternity entitlements as well as your obligations to your employer.

USING COMPLEMENTARY THERAPIES

There are a number of gentle ways of nurturing more positive, stress-free surroundings.

• The flower remedy yarrow special formula may be of benefit if you are exposed to environmental stresses during pregnancy, including radiation or any form of toxicity. It is especially useful if you have to travel, particularly by air. (You should avoid flying during the first trimester, especially if you have a history of miscarriage.) This remedy can be taken internally but also applied topically to the abdomen.

• Quartz crystals may be of benefit around the home and workplace. Place crystals near your computer, for example, if you spend a lot of time in front of one. Amber crystals, citrine and tourmaline are believed to offer some protection from electromagnetic fields and radiation. A bright crystal hung above the entrance to a home is believed to encourage *qi* into the building.

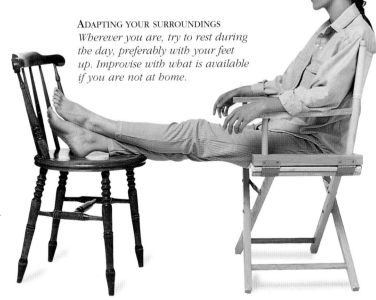

ADAPTING YOUR SURROUNDINGS
Wherever you are, try to rest during the day, preferably with your feet up. Improvise with what is available if you are not at home.

Antenatal Checks

ALL PREGNANT WOMEN ARE MONITORED routinely throughout their pregnancy at antenatal visits to a midwife or doctor. A range of tests may be recommended in order to detect foetal abnormalities, depending on the mother's medical or family history, experience in previous pregnancies, or her age.

ROUTINE TESTS

At your first antenatal visit, a midwife will take your medical history and advise you about diet, smoking and drinking alcohol. She will take a blood sample and feel your abdomen. At this and subsequent visits, your blood pressure will be checked and urine tested. It depends on your hospital, but appointments are usually every four weeks until week 28, then every two weeks until week 36, and then weekly. All working women are entitled to be paid during antenatal visits.

BLOOD & URINE TESTS

Blood tests check blood group, haemoglobin levels (to see if you are anaemic) and immunity to rubella (if you are not

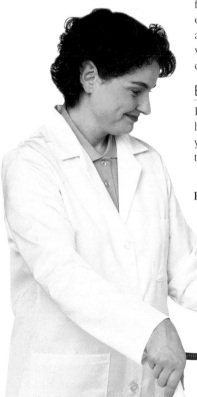

FOETAL HEARTBEAT
Listening to the foetal heartbeat for the first time can be very reassuring and reinforces the bond with your baby.

immune you will be offered a postnatal vaccination). They also test for syphilis, diabetes, hepatitis and your rhesus status. A rhesus negative mother with a rhesus positive baby will be given "anti-D" immunization at 28 weeks and after the birth. Rhesus disease may otherwise affect subsequent rhesus-positive children as the mother produces anti-rhesus positive antibodies. The blood-pressure reading taken at your first antenatal visit will be the one that every subsequent reading is measured against, so try to be as relaxed as possible. It is normal for your blood pressure to rise a little in late pregnancy. Urine is checked for ketones (which reduce the efficiency of oxygen transportation in the

ANTENATAL CHECKS

TRANSVAGINAL SCAN	ADVANTAGES *results are instant.*
Carried out from 5–6 weeks. A probe is inserted into the vagina giving a clear view of the growing baby.	DISADVANTAGES *baby exposed to high-frequency sound.*
CVS (CHORIONIC VILLUS SAMPLING)	ADVANTAGES *very accurate and preliminary results within 48 hours.*
Detects chromosomal and genetic disorders such as Down's syndrome and sickle-cell anaemia. A tube is inserted into the uterus at 8–12 weeks and cells taken from placental tissue surrounding the embryo.	DISADVANTAGES *risk of miscarriage (roughly one in 100).*
NUCHAL TEST	ADVANTAGES *non invasive and no risk of miscarriage.*
Non-invasive ultrasound scan carried out at 12 weeks to detect chromosomal disorders. "Nuchal" means neck: the scan checks for abnormal thickness in the fold at the back of the baby's neck. When combined with a blood test, the nuchal test is 80–90 per cent in accurate in predicting Down's syndrome.	DISADVANTAGES *none.*
AFP (ALPHA-FETOPROTEIN TEST)	ADVANTAGES *non-invasive with no side effects.*
Blood test that checks blood protein levels and detects neurological problems such as spina bifida or hydrocephalus. Carried out at 15–18 weeks. Accuracy is not good: high and low levels of alpha-fetoprotein can be found in women carrying perfectly normal babies and those who are very nauseous. Results take about 10 days.	DISADVANTAGES *only 50 per cent accurate; false-positive rate of 5–10 per cent.*
AMNIOCENTESIS	ADVANTAGES *very accurate (about 90 per cent); reveals baby's sex (important with some disorders).*
Sample of amniotic fluid taken under local anaesthetic through the abdominal wall at 16–18 weeks. Cells are tested for many disorders, including Down's syndrome. Results in 2–3 weeks.	DISADVANTAGES *risk of miscarriage (less than one in 100); discomfort; possible side effects (bleeding, infection); screens few defects.*
TRIPLE/QUADRUPLE/LEEDS/BART'S TESTS	ADVANTAGES *no risk of miscarriage.*
Combination of blood tests to assess risk of chromosomal defects or problems such as anencephaly (absence of a brain) or spina bifida.	DISADVANTAGES *accuracy between 60 and 80 per cent.*

blood), protein (which might indicate pre-eclampsia or an infection) and sugar. A glucose tolerance test (GTT) may be necessary to check for diabetes.

ULTRASOUND SCANNING

This is routine at 16–18 weeks. High-pitched sound waves are reflected back off the baby and reproduced electronically on a screen as an image. It confirms dates and multiple pregnancies, detects certain abnormalities and checks the position of the placenta. A scan is painless and there is no risk of miscarriage.

SPECIAL TESTS

You need to think long and hard about special antenatal tests (*see above*). Most of them are not obligatory. Make sure that you understand exactly what you are being offered and why, and if there will be any risk to your baby. Explore any alternatives before making a decision. You should consider that often your only option, should the results of any tests be positive, will be whether or not to terminate the pregnancy. Support and counselling will be on hand, however, in case of such an eventuality.

Out-of-the-ordinary Pregnancies

CERTAIN KINDS OF PREGNANCY are believed to put the foetus at a higher risk than normal. If you have any complications whatsoever, you will be monitored closely by medical professionals throughout your pregnancy. You will need to pay particular attention to your nutrition and other aspects of your lifestyle.

KEY TIPS

Rest as much as possible

✳

Give up work early

✳

Ensure that your diet includes good intakes of essential nutrients

✳

Report physical changes/symptoms

MULTIPLE PREGNANCIES

More women are giving birth to twins or triplets as a result of fertility treatment. A multiple pregnancy is not high-risk as such, but you are unlikely to go to term and, because of the possibility of complications during the birth, you will be advised against a home birth. You are also more likely to experience minor ailments such as morning sickness, heartburn, backache, sleeplessness, fatigue and raised blood pressure (*see pages 36–43, 54–67 and 78–91*). Plenty of rest and a good diet make good foundations for a multiple pregnancy. Great demands are made on your stores of iron and folate, for example, if you are carrying more than one baby so you could easily become anaemic.

OLDER MOTHERS

Many more women are having babies later in life. The older you are, the more important diet and lifestyle become. You will generally be advised to give up work as early as you can, rest as much as you can (particularly between 5 pm and 7 pm – *see page 132*) and eat

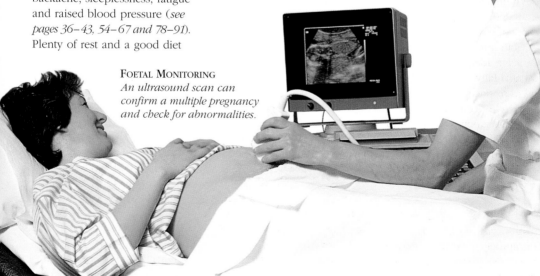

FOETAL MONITORING
An ultrasound scan can confirm a multiple pregnancy and check for abnormalities.

as healthy a diet as you can (*see pages 12–13*). This should include a good vitamin and mineral supplement.

IVF PREGNANCIES

Good preparation for in vitro fertilization (IVF) is essential. Women having this treatment tend to be older and to suffer what the Chinese regard as Kidney deficiency and weak *jing*, both of which can be corrected by acupuncture. Be sure to take time off work and rest completely at the time of egg transfer. Eat a diet rich in zinc and essential fatty acids, important for cell division and healthy cell membranes.

PREMATURE LABOUR

A premature labour is one that starts six weeks or more before your due date. If you went into labour early in a previous pregnancy, the chances are that you will do so again. Acupuncture may help if you have a history of premature birth but you need to start treatment in mid-pregnancy. Plenty of rest and good nutrition are both important. Make sure you have adequate supplies of essential fatty acids and zinc and iron, since deficiencies in these have been linked with premature labour. Watch out for symptoms of a urinary infection, which can cause premature labour, or low backache, which may indicate the start of labour.

DIABETES

Gestational diabetes develops during pregnancy and affects around five per cent of women who previously had no history of diabetes. This potentially serious condition usually develops during the second half of pregnancy and will be detected by routine antenatal urine tests. This condition will make you more prone to infections such as cystitis and thrush and to raised blood pressure. Induction or a Caesarean section may be recommended at 36 weeks. You will be closely monitored by your midwife or obstetrician and a nutritionist. Controlling diabetes by dietary measures requires care and self-discipline: eat little and often, choose your food carefully (*see below*) and limit alcohol consumption. Constitutional homeopathic treatment (*see pages 148–9*), for which you will need to consult a practitioner, may help .

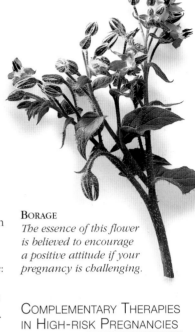

BORAGE
The essence of this flower is believed to encourage a positive attitude if your pregnancy is challenging.

COMPLEMENTARY THERAPIES IN HIGH-RISK PREGNANCIES

If your pregnancy is at all high-risk, it is important that any complementary therapy you consider is taken in conjunction with conventional treatment and advice from your midwife and doctor and in their full knowledge. Consult qualified complementary practitioners and inform them of your condition. Flower remedies are gentle and may be of help to a number of conditions. Angelica is generally beneficial in early pregnancy if you have a history of miscarriage; borage is said to lift the spirits if circumstances surrounding your pregnancy are difficult; California wild rose is generally useful for difficult pregnancies; gentian is good for coping with setbacks during pregnancy; mariposa lily helps to encourage a positive outlook and is useful at all stages of pregnancy; while tiger lily promotes a successful pregnancy in older women.

REDUCING SUGAR INTAKE

If you have sugar in your urine, you should avoid certain foods. You can eat as much as you like of others.

FOODS TO AVOID
• Sugar, fizzy drinks, cordials and squashes, biscuits and cakes, sweet puddings and some canned foods
• Fatty foods
• Salt and salty foods
• Highly processed foods

FOODS TO EAT FREELY
• Starchy foods such as bread, pasta, rice, noodles and cereals
• Fruit and vegetables
• Pulses
• Low-fat alternatives

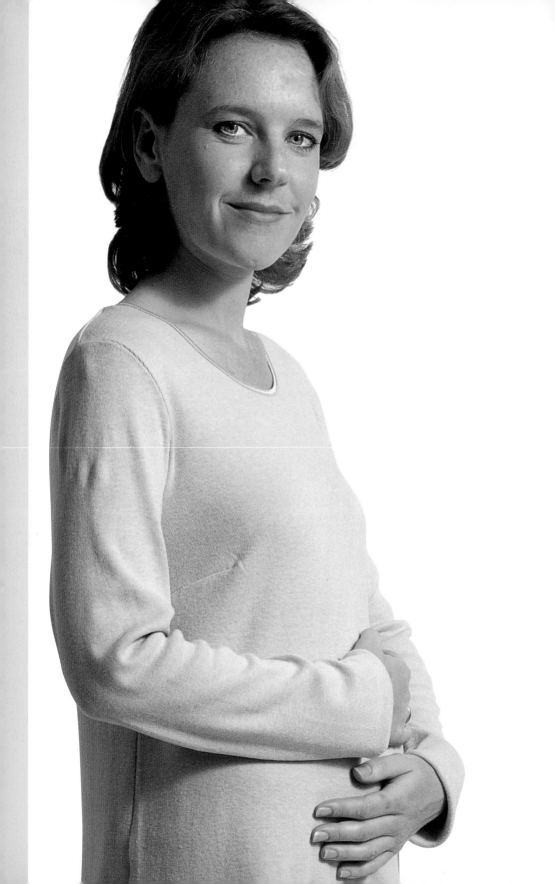

THE FIRST THREE MONTHS OF PREGNANCY are exciting but they can also give rise to anxiety. You and your partner may feel that it is too early to share your news with family and friends, but you are having to come to terms with great changes, not only to your body but also to both your lives. You will need time to adjust to the

The first trimester

idea of parenthood, and with this will come emotional highs and lows. This chapter addresses some of your natural anxieties, offers advice on how to keep as well as possible in terms of diet and exercise, and suggests how to deal with minor ailments that may affect you during this early stage of pregnancy.

FIRST TRIMESTER

Development of Mother & Baby

THE DEVELOPMENT OF A BABY TAKES 38 WEEKS from conception (40 weeks of pregnancy is calculated from the first day of your last menstrual period). By the third week after conception, you may realize that your period is late and suspect that you are pregnant.

> ## KEY TIPS
>
> *Consider antenatal tests carefully: they are not compulsory*
>
> *✳*
>
> *Eat little and often if you are feeling nauseous*
>
> *✳*
>
> *Rest if you feel tired*
>
> *✳*
>
> *Accept that it may take time to adjust to being pregnant*

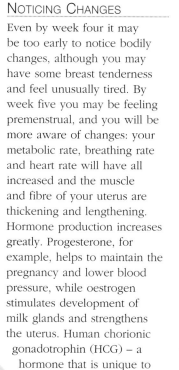

NOTICING CHANGES

Even by week four it may be too early to notice bodily changes, although you may have some breast tenderness and feel unusually tired. By week five you may be feeling premenstrual, and you will be more aware of changes: your metabolic rate, breathing rate and heart rate will have all increased and the muscle and fibre of your uterus are thickening and lengthening. Hormone production increases greatly. Progesterone, for example, helps to maintain the pregnancy and lower blood pressure, while oestrogen stimulates development of milk glands and strengthens the uterus. Human chorionic gonadotrophin (HCG) – a hormone that is unique to pregnancy – is produced by the placenta.

EARLY DAYS
There will be few outward signs of the great changes occurring within your body during the first 12 weeks.

Hormonal changes may cause great emotional highs and lows as well as nausea and sickness.

MAKING PLANS

By week six your pregnancy will have been confirmed. Contact your midwife or doctor and arrange for your first visit to an antenatal clinic between weeks eight and 12. Also make an appointment to see your dentist to maintain healthy teeth and gums. You will be aware of the speeding up of your metabolism. You may feel drained – as if someone has "pulled the plug". By about week eight you may experience mild abdominal pains as your uterus starts to stretch. If you suffer severe abdominal pain, see your doctor immediately. By week nine you should be thinking about antenatal tests. There are several screening and diagnostic tests to detect foetal abnormalities, but consider the implications of a positive result (*see page 23*). By week 12 the uterus is starting to move out of the pelvis, becoming an abdominal organ, and the heart is pumping extra blood.

THE BABY'S DEVELOPMENT

WEEK 1 After fertilization, the sperm and ovum nuclei fuse to form a zygote. This starts to divide as it travels to the uterus.

WEEK 2 After six or seven days, the cell mass develops a hollow cavity and is now called a blastocyst. By the tenth day it becomes embedded in the endometrium.

WEEK 3 The blastocyst is the size of a pinhead but is multiplying fast. The inner cells of the cavity develop into the embryo.

WEEK 4 The baby is about 2 mm ($\frac{1}{16}$ in) in length and weighs less than 1 gm ($\frac{3}{100}$ oz). Its body tissues are forming from three embryonic layers: the hair, nails, mammary glands, teeth enamel, inner ear and lenses for the eyes from one layer; the nervous system, retina, pituitary gland, muscle, cartilage, bones, blood and lymph cells from another; and lungs, trachea, liver, pancreas and bladder from a third.

WEEK 5 The heart has started to develop: it now has four chambers. The roof palate of the mouth is forming.

WEEK 6 The cluster of cells is becoming an embryo, roughly the size of a fingertip. The heart is beating at 180 beats a minute, more than twice as fast as yours. Eyelids, ears, and the beginnings of hands and feet are forming. The shape of the head and the curve of the spine are discernible.

WEEK 7 The embryo has quadrupled in size and the nervous system is developing well. The baby is starting to move its body, arms and legs. These movements can be detected by a monitor, but you will not be able to feel them. The lungs, liver and kidneys are starting to develop.

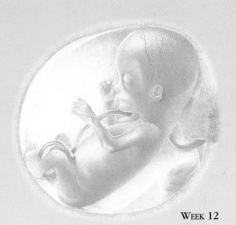

WEEK 12

WEEK 8 About 2.5 cm (1 in) in length, the embryo has now evolved into a foetus. Its brain is developing rapidly, and the umbilical cord has formed. Ears are beginning to develop and the mouth is able to open and close.

WEEK 9 The baby is now 4 cm ($1\frac{1}{2}$ in) in length and can wriggle slightly. The digestive and nervous systems are developing fast and the brain is four times larger than it was four weeks ago.

WEEK 10 The nervous system has matured enough for the baby to move about more. All the organs plus the sack of amniotic fluid have been formed and the baby is now recognizable as a human being.

WEEK 11 The liver takes over the manufacture of red blood cells and the kidneys are functioning. The baby is about 5 cm (2 in) long and growing rapidly. It has a completely formed face. The head is growing to accommodate the brain.

WEEK 12 Your baby is fully formed, although, at just 6 cm ($2\frac{1}{2}$ in) long, there is a lot of growing still to do. Its nails and hair are starting to grow, its jaw has 32 little teeth buds, and it is starting to suck. Internal sex organs have formed.

Nutrition for Mother & Baby

THE FIRST THREE MONTHS OF PREGNANCY are in many ways the most crucial for your baby's healthy development. A poor diet may affect the formation of organs and the development of body systems, as well as leading to a reduced birth weight. Certain vitamins and minerals are particularly important.

KEY TIPS

Eat little and often if you are feeling nauseous

✳

Include plenty of iron-rich foods in your diet

✳

Take a folic acid supplement

FUELLING DEVELOPMENT

Nutrition prior to conception is extremely important (*see pages 10–13*). This, in effect, extends into pregnancy, in that many women do not discover that they are pregnant until four or five weeks after conception. By this time many important developments have already occurred in the embryo. By the end of 12 weeks, a baby is fully formed, and the framework for all the organs, limbs, muscles, and bones is already in place (*see pages 29*).

KEY NUTRIENTS

Of the key food types, protein is needed in large amounts by the mother for building and repairing cells, muscles, organs, tissues and hair, and for enzyme production. At least half the calories should come from carbohydrates, mainly in the form of starch. Of the key nutrients needed at this time, folate and iron are vitally important. Folate is a B vitamin used for cell division, red blood cell formation, and development of the baby's nervous system. Since the neural tube forms in the fourth week of gestation, you should boost folate supplies by taking a folic acid supplement before you conceive to help to prevent defects such as spina bifida. Folate levels are difficult to maintain from food alone so you may need to continue the supplement. Iron is found in haemoglobin, and is needed to transport oxygen and carbon dioxide, to make enzymes and to generate energy. The demand for iron increases in pregnancy due to an increase in blood volume in an expectant woman and the development of the placenta.

KEY DAILY DIETARY CONSTITUENTS

6 servings of grains
5 servings of vegetables
2 servings of lean meat, fish or pulses
2 servings of folic-acid-rich foods
2 servings of calcium-rich foods
Plenty of filtered or mineral water

SUMMER VEGETABLES
Roasted red and yellow peppers, tomatoes, cucumber, anchovies and eggs provide a substantial main-course salad dish.

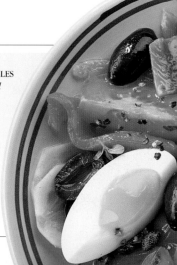

ESSENTIAL DIETARY NUTRIENTS

VITAMINS & MINERALS	FOR MOTHER	FOR BABY
VITAMIN A Some of your intake of beta carotene may be converted into vitamin A.	*For its anti-oxidant properties and to fight infection.*	*For cell differentiation, eye development, formation of healthy cell membranes.*
B VITAMINS You do not need to increase intakes unless you are adolescent, carrying twins or at risk of diabetes.	*B^2 and B^6 to balance hormones; B^2 and B^5 for energy; B^6 to improve metabolism.*	*B^{12} for nervous system; B^6 for healthy immune system and brain development.*
OTHER VITAMINS The need for vitamin D increases in pregnancy, and also for vitamin E if consumption of polyunsaturated fats is high.	*C for iron absorption and hormone production; D to absorb and utilize calcium.*	*D for healthy bones; E for the developing heart.*
FOLATE	*See Key Nutrients, opposite.*	*See Key Nutrients, opposite.*
IRON	*See Key Nutrients, opposite.*	*See Key Nutrients, opposite.*
CALCIUM The foetus accumulates calcium rapidly during the first trimester.	*For healthy bones and teeth.*	*For muscle contraction and nerve transmission.*
ZINC Essential throughout pregnancy.	*For production of hormones.*	*For cell reproduction and growth; to prevent low birth weight.*
OTHER MINERALS Good iodine levels are needed prior to conception. Chromium may prevent nausea. Magnesium may prevent raised blood pressure.	*Manganese and chromium for blood sugar regulation; manganese and magnesium for hormone balance and energy production.*	*Manganese for prevention of foetal malformations; iodine to prevent hyperthyroidism.*

SUGGESTED MEAL PLAN

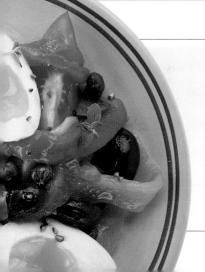

BREAKFAST
Oatflake cereal with sesame seeds, banana, pear and milk

MIDMORNING SNACK
Apple, oatcake and slice of Cheddar cheese

LUNCH
Mackerel with watercress, grated carrot and tomato; wholemeal bread and butter; an orange

AFTERNOON SNACK
Dried figs and almonds

DINNER
Lamb and black-eyed bean casserole, potatoes, carrots and broccoli

BEDTIME SNACK
Pure fruit blueberry jam with wholemeal bread and butter

Exercise Plan

HUGE EMOTIONAL AND PHYSICAL CHANGES take place during the early months of pregnancy. Some women worry about their level of fitness and want to rush straight into an exercise programme, while others struggle to cope with the emotional roller-coaster and the fatigue typical of early pregnancy.

KEY TIPS

Stop exercising if you experience serious discomfort or pain

✳

Do not over-exert yourself

✳

Do not get overheated

✳

Set yourself realistic targets

WARMING UP & COOLING DOWN

IT IS IMPORTANT *to warm up when you start exercising. The aim of a warm-up is to mobilize major joints – by means of static stretches – then to move the joints to warm them up. This is* *followed by aerobic exercise that raises the pulse further and strengthens the muscles. You should then cool down, stretching out muscles that have been worked. Finally, relax the body.*

GENERAL GUIDELINES

You should at all times be aware of general guidelines relating to exercise during pregnancy (*see pages 18–19*).

MOBILIZING JOINTS

Work through the body, starting from the top.

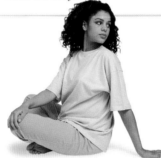

• **Head and neck** Sitting cross-legged, turn the head slowly and smoothly from side to side 6–8 times. Then, lower the ear towards the shoulder and lift it back up. Repeat 6–8 times on each side. Turn the head to one side and slowly sweep the chin across the chest to the other side. Repeat 6–8 times on each side.

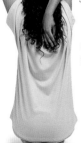

• **Shoulders and arms** Lift the right shoulder and lower, then the left. Repeat 6–8 times. Then, pull both shoulders forward, lift and push back. Do this 6–8 times, then repeat rotating forwards. Finally, kneel and sit on your heels. Stretch the right arm up and bend it so that your hand is behind your back. Use the left hand to push the elbow gently backwards to increase the stretch (*see left*). Repeat with the left arm.

• **Spine and pelvis** Sit with legs crossed, back straight and neck stretched slightly upwards. Breathing out, turn the upper body to the right, placing your right hand behind you for stability (*see centre left*). Put the left hand on the right knee and use it to push your body slightly further round. Repeat to the left. Then, stand with feet hip-width apart, knees soft, and hips and feet facing forwards. Rotate the upper body slowly in each direction several times. Do the same with the hips. Finally, tucking the bottom under and tilting the pelvis upwards, tighten the abdominal muscles.

• **Hips and legs** Stand with feet slightly wider than hip-width apart, knees soft, bottom tucked under and pelvis tilted upwards. Lift the right hip and hold for five seconds. Repeat 6–8 times, then with the left hip. Sitting with legs out and leaning on the arms for support, bend each leg and straighten it several times (*see below*).

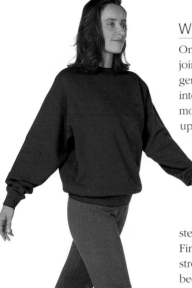

MARCHING
Walking briskly will increase your heart rate, improving cardiovascular function.

WORKING HARDER

Once you have mobilized the joints, combine two or three gentle, low-impact aerobic steps into a five-minute programme to move the joints and warm them up and raise the pulse slightly. This might include marching backwards and forwards, marching on the spot with knee-lifts, side-steps with half-squats and transfer-of-weight steps such as hamstring curls. Finally in the warm-up, gently stretch out muscles that have been worked to ease tension out of them. Next, proceed to aerobic work to maintain or improve your stamina and cardiovascular function, increase oxygen supply to all parts of the body and improve body awareness. While not raising your fitness level, this part of your exercise programme will equip you to deal with the physical demands of pregnancy and labour. Use the same steps as before, just make them more dynamic, and combine several into a 15-minute programme.

• **Hamstring curls** Step on to the right foot, bending the left leg and bringing the left foot up towards the bottom. Swing your arms from side to side. Repeat, stepping to the left.

MUSCLE STRENGTH & ENDURANCE

Pregnant women should target specific muscles to improve posture and prepare them for labour and life beyond the birth. So, after your aerobic work, do exercises to strengthen the upper body, such as pec-decks and box-position press-ups, to help with bending and lifting, for example. Exercises for the lower body include side leg-lifts or static half-squats on the spot. Other exercises may help to relieve aches and pains (*see below*). Stretch out all muscles used in a final cool-down.

LOWER BACK STRETCHES

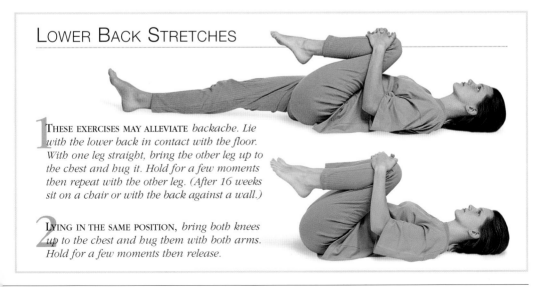

1 THESE EXERCISES MAY ALLEVIATE *backache. Lie with the lower back in contact with the floor. With one leg straight, bring the other leg up to the chest and hug it. Hold for a few moments then repeat with the other leg. (After 16 weeks sit on a chair or with the back against a wall.)*

2 LYING IN THE SAME POSITION, *bring both knees up to the chest and hug them with both arms. Hold for a few moments then release.*

FIRST TRIMESTER

Five-point Action Plan

THE FIRST THREE MONTHS of pregnancy are an exciting but possibly also a nerve-wracking time, whether your baby is planned or a surprise. During these first few weeks, you will be coming to terms not only with the physical changes to your body but with the impact that a new baby is going to have on your life. The following advice may be helpful.

GET ENOUGH SLEEP

A good night's sleep is the best foundation on which to start each day. You may find yourself in bed by 8 pm each evening, as you respond to your body's needs. Promote restful sleep by eating a light supper at the end of the day so as not to overload your digestive system before you go to bed. Try and put your feet up during the day and catnap during the afternoon, if work or other children permit.

TAKE TIME TO ADJUST

You will experience emotional highs and lows, and you may feel more exhausted than ever before. You will have many decisions to make: when to tell people your news; when to stop work; what childcare provisions need to be made. Many people prefer to keep their news a secret for the first three months, waiting until they are more confident about their pregnancy. Do not rush decisions: take time to adjust and make plans.

EXERCISE SENSIBLY

Do not force yourself to exercise at this stage of pregnancy if you do not feel like it. Gentle forms of exercise such as walking, stretching and swimming are preferable to a strenuous work-out in the gym. More research is needed on the possible effects of the mother's increased body temperature as a result of exertion on the formation of her baby's vital organs during the first three months. Do not over-exert yourself or get overheated.

IMPROVE YOUR DIET

Take a good look at what you eat. Vitamins and minerals are often eliminated by modern methods of cultivation, food processing and cooking. The chances are that you lack the full complement of nutrients needed while your baby's organs are forming. Try to eat fresh organic food, take a good all-round multivitamin and a folic acid supplement, and avoid alcohol, tea, coffee and highly processed foods.

PREPARE MENTALLY

Take time out each day to be quiet and calm and to reflect upon what is happening to you and how your life is changing. Apart from all the practical considerations that you need to give thought to, it is also important to start to form a relationship with your unborn baby by visualizing the child. Listen to music if it helps to soothe your mind and relax your body.

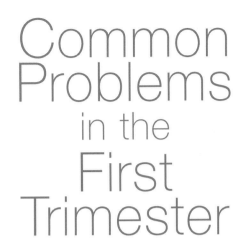

Common Problems in the First Trimester

THIS CAN BE AN ANXIOUS TIME, when you are not yet fully confident about your pregnancy. You may also feel very drained of energy and emotion. The following pages will help you to deal with some of the minor ailments that are common in early pregnancy.

FIRST TRIMESTER

Morning Sickness

ABOUT HALF OF PREGNANT WOMEN experience morning sickness. It is most likely to affect those with nutritional deficiencies. The development of the placenta and associated hormone levels, which peak at 9–10 weeks, may be responsible, but vomiting can also be the body's way of eliminating toxins.

SYMPTOMS

Nausea and vomiting
*
Excessive salivation
*
Disinclination to eat
*
Side effect: fatigue

DIET & NUTRITION

Eat foods that appeal to you and are easy to prepare, and eat frequently as this stabilizes blood sugar levels. Your need for vitamins B6 and B12, folic acid, iron and zinc increases in pregnancy. Nausea is linked with B6 and zinc deficiencies in particular. If you vomit a lot you may also develop a magnesium deficiency. Vitamin and mineral supplements are helpful but are difficult to take if you feel very sick. Eat the following foods to replenish vitamin and mineral levels:

* Wholemeal bread, chickpeas, seeds, hazelnuts and raisins, which are good sources of vitamin B6.
* Milk, yogurt and white fish, which contain vitamin B12.
* Green leafy vegetables, yeast extract, fortified breakfast cereals, nuts and pulses for folic acid.
* Broccoli, apricots and sardines to raise iron levels.
* Poultry, lean meat, sunflower seeds, wholemeal bread and wheatgerm to replenish zinc.
* Nuts, wholegrains, apricots and tofu for magnesium.

See pages 30–1 for further information

EASING NAUSEA
Try this gentle breathing exercise before each meal. Place one hand on your stomach and the other hand on your chest and focus on your stomach as you breathe deeply for five minutes.

KEY TIPS

Rest as much as possible
*
Eat what your body tells you to and drink plenty of water
*
Eat small, frequent meals
*
Avoid fatty or spicy foods
*
Keep a snack by your bed to eat before getting up in the morning

CAUTIONS

Drink plenty of fluids to avoid dehydration, signs of which include rapid pulse, furry tongue, bad-smelling breath and passing little urine. If you are experiencing persistent vomiting (*see pages 38–9*), consult your doctor.

COMPLEMENTARY TREATMENTS

Before using a complementary treatment, please read any **Cautions** and the relevant page references

ACUPUNCTURE

Needles are inserted into acupoints on your body, depending on the history and nature of your morning sickness. Between four and six weekly treatments may be needed.

✳ A practitioner may insert fine needles into the Pericardium 6 acupoint, located on your forearm, for between 15 and 20 minutes.

See pages 134–5 for further information

ACUPRESSURE

Based on the same Chinese principles as acupuncture – that sickness arises due to a blockage of *qi* – a practitioner balances *qi* by stimulating acupoints. Try these self-help measures:

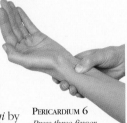

PERICARDIUM 6
Press three finger-widths from the wrist, between both tendons.

✳ Stimulate the Pericardium 6 acupoint on your forearm to try to relieve nausea. Do this for ten minutes four times a day.

✳ Wear special acumagnets on the same acupoint day and night, since this can sometimes bring relief.

See page 136 for further information

REFLEXOLOGY

Nausea and sickness may respond to reflexology, especially in combination with other complementary treatments such as

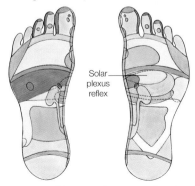

Solar plexus reflex

acupuncture, shiatsu or homeopathy. A reflexologist will gently massage the solar

plexus zone on the sole of the left foot that is linked to the relief of nausea.

See pages 140–1 for further information

YOGA & MEDITATION

Yoga and meditation can ease nausea by relaxing the diaphragm. To encourage relaxation, a yoga practitioner teaches a series of postures (*asanas*) that aim to integrate mind and body, so relieving tension.

✳ If any thoughts intrude during meditation, simply concentrate on the sensation of breathing.

See pages 142–3 for further information

WESTERN HERBALISM

Ginger is a key herb used in the treatment of morning sickness. It is rich in zinc, therefore helping to combat deficiency – a possible cause of nausea. It has been shown in clinical trials to reduce nausea and vomiting attacks.

✳ Eat ginger in any form, such as crystallized ginger or ginger biscuits, or, preferably, drink ginger tea. Infuse 5 g (1 tsp) grated ginger root in a cup of freshly boiled water for five minutes. Drink a cup two or three times a day or sip it frequently throughout the day.

✳ Other herbal teas can help, including chamomile, fennel, spearmint or peppermint. Drink a cup three times a day. Alternatively, any of these teas can be made into ice-cubes and sucked.

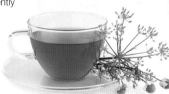

CHAMOMILE AND FENNEL
These gentle, soothing teas relieve sickness.

See pages 150–1 for further information

HOMEOPATHY

Try one of the following homeopathic self-help remedies, depending on your symptoms.

✳ For morning sickness with irritability, *Nux vomica 6c*.

✳ For inability to keep anything down but nausea not relieved by vomiting, *Ipecac. 6c*.

✳ For evening sickness and tearfulness, *Pulsatilla 6c*.

See pages 148–9 for dosage and further information

FIRST TRIMESTER

Hyperemesis

SEVERE VOMITING during pregnancy affects one in 100 women. Although not very common, it may well recur in subsequent pregnancies. Hyperemesis causes dehydration and upsets nutritional balance, and you may require hospitalization. Eating the right foods in the months prior to conception may help to prevent this condition.

SYMPTOMS

Inability to keep food down and severe, repeated vomiting

❋

Dehydration

❋

Side effect: depression and a feeling of isolation

PERICARDIUM 6
Your acupuncturist may also use this acupoint on the forearm to relieve nausea and sickness (see opposite).

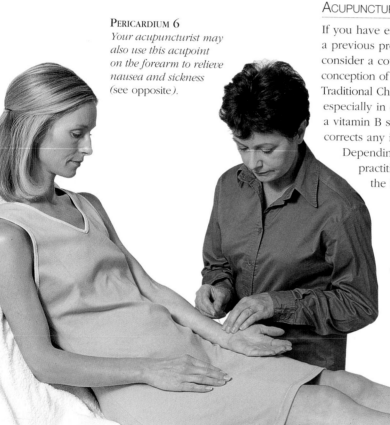

ACUPUNCTURE

If you have experienced hyperemesis in a previous pregnancy, you may wish to consider a course of acupuncture prior to conception of your next baby. According to Traditional Chinese Medicine, acupuncture, especially in conjunction with zinc and a vitamin B supplement (*see opposite*), corrects any imbalances in pregnancy. Depending on your symptoms, a practitioner will stimulate points on the Stomach or Liver meridians.

❋ An acupuncturist will insert fine needles and leave them in place for 15–20 minutes.

See pages 134–5 for further information

KEY TIPS

Rest as much as possible
❋
Get up slowly and avoid sudden movements
❋
Drink plenty of fluids
❋
Eat small, frequent snacks
❋
Avoid bad smells
❋
Have a bedtime snack to prevent blood sugar levels dropping at night

CAUTION

If you are experiencing persistent vomiting, watch for signs of dehydration (*see page 36*), continue to drink plenty of fluids and consult your doctor.

COMPLEMENTARY TREATMENTS

Before using a complementary treatment, please read any **Cautions** and the relevant page references

ACUPRESSURE

The Stomach and Liver meridians are often used in the treatment of nausea. In addition, the Pericardium 6 acupoint, located three finger-widths down the arm from the wrist crease, between the tendons, may be pressed for ten minutes four times a day to bring relief.

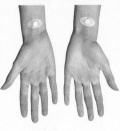

✳ For the same effect, place acumagnets so that they put pressure on the Pericardium 6 acupoint.

✳ If you are very sick, use a TENS machine (*see page 109*). Place a pad on each Pericardium 6 acupoint for 45 minutes twice a day.

ACUMAGNETS
Sticky-backed acumagnets are easy to put in place.

See page 136 for further information

CHIROPRACTIC

A chiropractor will manipulate your spine and joints in order to realign your body and improve digestive function. Studies have shown that this treatment can ease nausea.

See page 147 for further information

HYPNOTHERAPY

This treatment can help to alleviate stress and vomiting, but is only effective if you are receptive. Use a reputable practitioner who is recommended by the maternity services. A hypnotherapist may suggest self-help measures so that you can regulate the nausea at home.

See page 145 for further information

HOMEOPATHY

A homeopath will choose a remedy according to your symptoms. It might be:

✳ For sudden, spasmodic and severe vomiting, *Antim. tart. 6c.*

✳ For persistent vomiting that does not relieve the nausea, *Ipecac. 6c.*

See pages 148–9 for dosage and further information

AROMATHERAPY

You may find that burning essential oils such as lemon or bergamot in the room raises your spirits and relieves your nausea.

Caution: see page 153 for oils to avoid in pregnancy.

See pages 152–3 for further information

BERGAMOT
Fresh-smelling oil from the bergamot plant is uplifting.

FLOWER REMEDIES

Women with hyperemesis often feel anxious, tired and emotional. The following flower remedies may help to bring relief:

✳ Red chestnut if you are anxious about your baby.

✳ Crab apple for feelings of self-disgust.

✳ Chamomile for emotional upset.

See page 154 for further information

DIET & NUTRITION

The foetus can still obtain the nutrients it needs if you have hyperemesis, but try to eat the foods listed below. Bland carbohydrates, such as rice, baked potatoes, pasta and dry toast, however, may be the only foods you can tolerate. If you have had hyperemesis before, take a vitamin B[6] supplement before conceiving your next baby.

✳ Vitamin B[6] deficiency increases nausea. Eat bananas, chickpeas, wholemeal bread, brown rice and raisins.

✳ Pregnant women need extra zinc, and vegetarians often already lack zinc. Zinc-rich foods include ginger, poultry, lean meat, wholemeal bread and almonds.

✳ Magnesium is lost through vomiting, so eat plenty of nuts, wholegrains, wheatgerm and dried apricots.

✳ Potassium-rich foods, such as bananas, melons, raisins, figs and fruit juice, are essential after sickness.

See pages 30–1 for further information

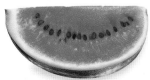

MELON
This fruit replenishes potassium, needed to redress fluid imbalance caused by vomiting.

Mouth Problems

HORMONAL CHANGES during pregnancy cause gums to thicken and soften, which may lead to tooth and gum problems. Gingivitis (inflamed gums) is common in the first half of pregnancy and can lead to bleeding gums and the loss of teeth. Cold sores on the lips are caused by the *herpes simplex* virus, and often appear if the immune system is weakened.

SYMPTOMS

Inflamed, sore and bleeding gums

✳

Blisters on the lips

✳

Unusual taste sensations

✳

Loose or aching teeth

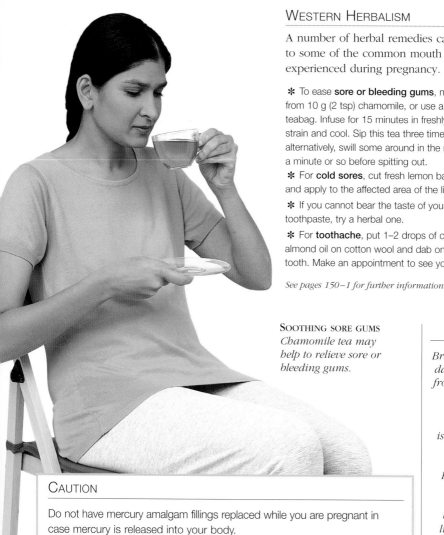

WESTERN HERBALISM

A number of herbal remedies can bring relief to some of the common mouth problems experienced during pregnancy.

✳ To ease **sore or bleeding gums**, make an infusion from 10 g (2 tsp) chamomile, or use a chamomile teabag. Infuse for 15 minutes in freshly boiled water, strain and cool. Sip this tea three times a day; alternatively, swill some around in the mouth for a minute or so before spitting out.

✳ For **cold sores**, cut fresh lemon balm leaves and apply to the affected area of the lips.

✳ If you cannot bear the taste of your usual toothpaste, try a herbal one.

✳ For **toothache**, put 1–2 drops of clove oil diluted in almond oil on cotton wool and dab on to the affected tooth. Make an appointment to see your dentist.

See pages 150–1 for further information

SOOTHING SORE GUMS
Chamomile tea may help to relieve sore or bleeding gums.

KEY TIPS

Brush your teeth twice a day, using short strokes from gum to tooth edge, and floss daily

✳

Follow a diet that is low in refined sugar and starch

✳

Have regular dental check-ups

✳

Use sunblock on the lips to help to prevent cold sores

CAUTION

Do not have mercury amalgam fillings replaced while you are pregnant in case mercury is released into your body.

COMPLEMENTARY TREATMENTS

Before using any complementary treatments, please read any **Cautions** and relevant page references

HOMEOPATHY

There are several homeopathic remedies that may be prescribed for ailments affecting the teeth, gums and lips. A homeopath can prescribe a constitutional remedy depending on your medical history and symptoms, or you can self-prescribe. Choose one of the following homeopathic remedies, depending to your specific symptoms:

✳ For bad breath and **spongy gums**, *Merc. sol. 6c.*

✳ For red, inflamed, and **swollen gums** that bleed easily, *Kreosotum 6c.*

✳ For **bleeding gums**, *Phosphorus 6c.*

✳ For **cold sores**, *Natrum mur. 6c.*

PHOSPHORUS
Phosphorus is specifically prescribed for gums that bleed when touched.

See pages 148–9 for dosage and further information

DIET & NUTRITION

A varied diet that includes plenty of fresh fruit and vegetables – particularly green leafy vegetables – wholegrains, seeds and nuts, fish and lean meat will provide teeth and gums with all the nutrients that they need to stay healthy, and will boost the immune system so that it can fend off viruses. Be sure to chew food thoroughly, since the manipulation of food in the mouth helps to massage gums and increase blood flow through them. Your body's calcium requirement increases more than three-fold during pregnancy as the baby uses it to form teeth and bones. If your diet contains insufficient calcium, your baby's development may be affected and your own teeth and bones may also suffer as a result. It is also essential to eat foods that are good sources of magnesium, since this mineral

assists the absorption of calcium to create strong bones. Regular exercise also increases the absorption of calcium, as does vitamin D, which is produced under the skin by the action of ultraviolet radiation from the sun. Twenty minutes' exposure to the sun each day is probably all that you need. Make sure that you follow these dietary guidelines:

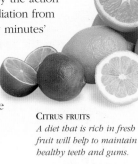

CITRUS FRUITS
A diet that is rich in fresh fruit will help to maintain healthy teeth and gums.

✳ Eat plenty of foods rich in vitamin C, which will maintain healthy gums and inhibit the development of **gingivitis**, **bleeding gums** and **cold sores**. Have five portions of fruit and vegetables daily; good choices are citrus fruit, blackcurrants, apples, apricots, cherries, Brussels sprouts, alfalfa, watercress and fresh parsley.

✳ Ensure that you receive sufficient calcium, which is essential for strong teeth, by eating parsley, watercress, nuts, sunflower seeds, eggs, low-fat milk, oily fish – for example, sardines and salmon – and chicken.

✳ Restrict intake of foods that inhibit calcium absorption. These include coffee, soft drinks, refined sugars, alcohol, protein (in excess) and salt.

✳ Eat foods that are rich in magnesium, which assists with calcium absorption. Good choices include dried apricots, wheatgerm, wholegrains, soya beans, cashew nuts, low-fat milk and yogurt.

✳ Include vitamin D-rich foods in your diet. Oily fish are by far the best source, but brown rice, eggs, milk, butter and margarine also contain vitamin D, which is needed to assist calcium absorption.

✳ Avoid eating large amounts of refined sugar and starch, since they can cause or exacerbate tooth decay while you have inflamed gums.

See pages 30–1 for further information

NUTS AND SEEDS
These are good sources of protein as well as of valuable nutrients such as magnesium.

FIRST TRIMESTER

Threatened Miscarriage

IT IS THOUGHT THAT ONE IN THREE PREGNANCIES miscarries; some women do not even realize they are pregnant. The causes of miscarriage include nutritional deficiencies, hormonal imbalance, infection, and auto-immune or chromosomal foetal disorders. Taking care prior to conception (*see pages 10–11*) is especially important if you have miscarried before.

SYMPTOMS

Backache

✳

Abdominal cramping pains resembling period pains

✳

Spots of blood or bleeding

ACUPUNCTURE

According to Traditional Chinese Medicine, the Kidneys are associated with reproduction. If there is weakness in the reproductive organs, an acupuncturist will aim to strengthen them by treating points on the Kidney meridian. The practitioner will take your case history, listen to your pulse and look at your tongue. Any sensations of heat or cold that you have are significant in cases of threatened miscarriage.

✳ The acupunture point that has traditionally been used in China in an attempt to prevent miscarriage is on the big toe (Sp 1). Moxa herb may be used to heat this point first.

See pages 134–5 for further information

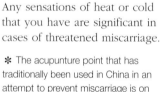

KEY TIPS

Avoid alcohol

✳

Avoid coffee, tea and cola drinks (caffeine has been linked to miscarriages)

✳

Avoid hot baths

✳

Do not smoke

✳

Get plenty of rest, especially between 5 pm and 7 pm
(see pages 132–3)

CAUTION

If you suspect that you might be about to miscarry, seek immediate medical attention. Therapies are only intended to complement, not replace, medical advice.

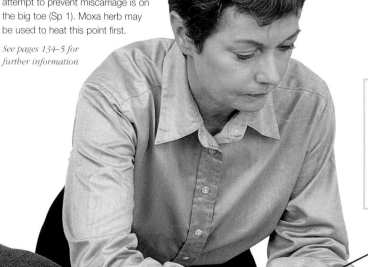

SPLEEN 1
A practitioner may heat the point on the big toe first – by lighting a small moxa cone with an akabani stick.

COMPLEMENTARY TREATMENTS

Before using a complementary treatment, please read any **Cautions** and the relevant page references

REIKI

Reiki treatment encourages a sense of deep relaxation, which may help if there is a risk of miscarriage. Practitioners believe that the body absorbs reiki energy much like a plant absorbs water. The energy flows to the source of the problem and acts as a catalyst for the body's own healing mechanisms.

See page 139 for further information

VISUALIZATION

Concentrate on your baby in the uterus, sending positive thoughts to it. Also try to visualize the colour blue, regarded as the colour of healing. In Traditional Chinese Medicine, blue is related to the water element and to the Kidneys, which are believed to be responsible for reproduction. Try sitting quietly for 15 minutes, visualizing an area of blue around your lower back and abdomen.

See page 143 for further information

VISUALIZATION
The power of thought may help to promote healing and therefore prevent miscarriage.

HOMEOPATHY

Depending on your symptoms, a homeopath may prescribe one of the following remedies to prevent a threatened miscarriage:

✳ For a steady loss of bright red blood, cramping abdominal pain, weakness and nausea, *Ipecac. 30c.*

✳ For stitching pains that begin in the back and spread to the front, *Kali carb. 30c.*

✳ For intermittent loss of dark red blood which is more profuse each time it occurs, *Pulsatilla 30c.*

See pages 148–9 for dosage and further information

WESTERN HERBALISM

False unicorn root has traditionally been given to prevent miscarriage, but this must only be taken under careful supervision by a medical herbalist. Ginger can also taken to prevent miscarriage, either added to food or as a tea. To make ginger tea, grate 5 g (1 tsp) fresh ginger and infuse in a cup of freshly boiled water.

See pages 150–1 for further information

AROMATHERAPY

Burn either lavender or lemon essential oil in a vaporizer to promote relaxation and help to reduce the threat of miscarriage.

Caution: see page 153 for oils to avoid in pregnancy.

See pages 152–3 for further information

FLOWER REMEDIES

Flower remedies may help to reduce anxiety about threatened miscarriage.

✳ Mimulus combats anxiety.
✳ White chestnut alleviates worry.
✳ Sweet chestnut eases despair.

See page 154 for further information

MIMULUS
The remedy made from this flower may dispel apprehension.

DIET & NUTRITION

Take multivitamins every day. Vitamin E may strengthen the placental link and reduce spotting, so take a supplement for two or three weeks or eat foods such as sweet potatoes and green leafy vegetables. Like vitamin E, selenium is an anti-oxidant and may help to prevent miscarriage. Take a supplement for three weeks or eat foods such as seafood or Brazil nuts.

✳ If you are bleeding, eat iron-rich foods, such as watercress and spinach, to prevent anaemia (*see also pages 56–7*).

See pages 30–1 for further information

GARLIC
Garlic is another source of the anti-oxidant selenium.

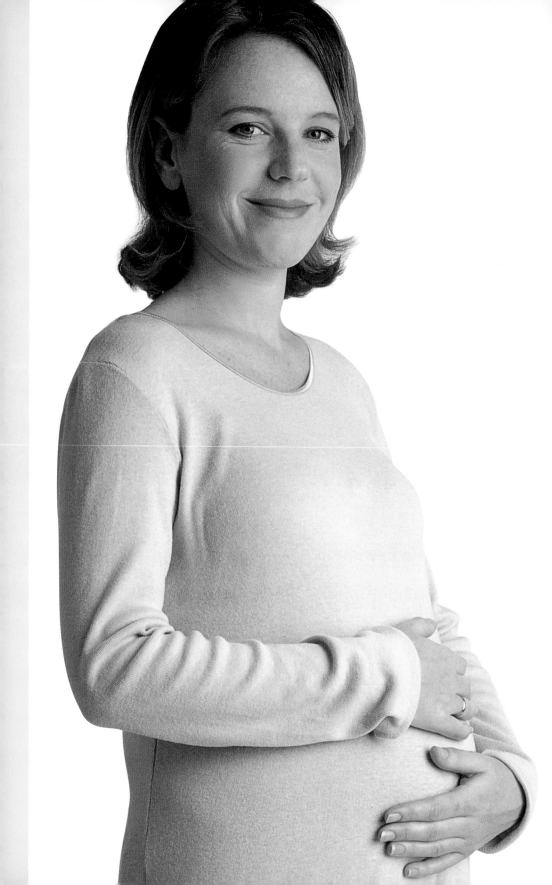

DURING THIS STAGE of your pregnancy you may well be "blooming", with shining hair and glowing skin. For many women this is the most enjoyable time: you should by now know the results of most antenatal tests and generally be feeling more confident and comfortable about your pregnancy. Sickness and exhaustion should

The second trimester

have lessened, while appetite and energy should have returned. There are some common problems and minor ailments that might affect you, however. This chapter offers practical advice to help you feel your best, both mentally and physically, and maintain a healthy diet and beneficial exercise programme.

Development of Mother & Baby

By NOW YOU SHOULD BE LESS TIRED and your appetite should start to improve. You will notice the first signs of a "bump" as the uterus begins to grow rapidly. You will be more aware of the baby as an individual, which may encourage strong nurturing feelings.

SECOND TRIMESTER

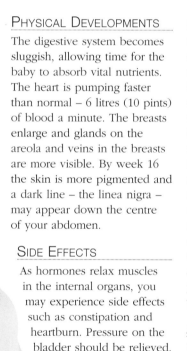

KEY TIPS

Book yourself in for antenatal classes at about 14 weeks, earlier for some, to avoid disappointment

✻

Have an ultrasound scan at about 19 weeks

✻

Take care to protect your back when bending and lifting

PHYSICAL DEVELOPMENTS

The digestive system becomes sluggish, allowing time for the baby to absorb vital nutrients. The heart is pumping faster than normal – 6 litres (10 pints) of blood a minute. The breasts enlarge and glands on the areola and veins in the breasts are more visible. By week 16 the skin is more pigmented and a dark line – the linea nigra – may appear down the centre of your abdomen.

SIDE EFFECTS

As hormones relax muscles in the internal organs, you may experience side effects such as constipation and heartburn. Pressure on the bladder should be relieved, however, as the growing uterus rises out of the pubic cavity. By week 18 your

LOOKING PREGNANT
You will have a noticeable "bump" and your waistline will have disappeared.

increased blood supply may cause nasal congestion and the occasional nosebleed. You may sweat more because of your increased metabolic rate. By week 17 you will be laying down fat: by week 24 you will be gaining 225–450 g (½–1 lb) a week in weight. This may increase further at week 27 as your baby puts on a growth spurt. The bump will be noticably bigger, and stretch marks may appear across your abdomen. The increased weight of the baby together with the softening affect of hormones on joints and ligaments will alter your sense of gravity.

AWARENESS OF BABY

By week 16 you may be aware of a "quickening" – the baby's first tangible movements. This feels like a slight fluttering or bubbling in your abdomen. By week 20, the baby's movements will be obvious. A couple of weeks later you will be able to detect cycles of activity and sleep. You may even be able to detect the baby's hiccups. By week 24, the baby may move when you start to speak.

THE BABY'S DEVELOPMENT

WEEK 13 The body is growing rapidly. The placenta now maintains the pregnancy, supplying nutrients and oxygen.

WEEK 14 The baby is aware of noise and light and responds to touch. Limbs are fully formed. Kidneys are beginning to function: the baby swallows amniotic fluid, rather than absorbing it through the skin, and excretes it. Few infections cross the placenta now.

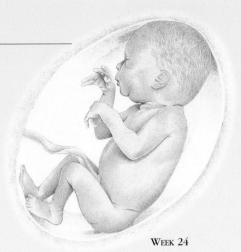

WEEK 24

WEEK 15 The body is growing faster than the head and movements are more vigorous. The bones still consist of soft cartilage but are beginning to ossify. Brain cells are increasing by 250,000 a minute.

WEEK 16 Facial features are looking more human. Fine hair (lanugo) is forming all over the body. Nerves are beginning to develop myelin sheaths, which will speed up neural connections.

WEEK 17 The baby measures about 18 cm (7 in) in length and weighs about 170 g (6 oz). The face can frown and squint; eyelashes and eyebrows are developing.

WEEK 18 The baby is practising breathing, taking amniotic fluid into the lungs and "breathing" it out again. It may have started to suck its thumb.

WEEK 19 Brain cells are continuing to multiply at an astonishing rate: between 50,000 and 100,000 a minute. The spinal cord is starting to thicken.

WEEK 20 The baby is roughly half as long as it will be at birth. Hair is growing on the head. Growth now slows, allowing body systems to mature.

WEEK 21 Taste buds have developed. The baby is starting to drink large amounts of ammiotic fluid.

WEEK 22 Ears are fully formed. The baby may be able to learn and respond to sounds and voices. Music may stimulate brain-cell activity.

WEEK 23 Limbs are well developed and hands are able to grip. You will be able to identify different parts of the baby's body through the abdominal wall.

WEEK 24 Eyes can open. The baby can identify voices. Air sacs in the lungs are fully formed though, if born now, the baby would have severe breathing difficulties. All major organs are formed. Heart rate has dropped and is recordable. Skin is translucent and blood vessels clearly visible through it.

WEEK 25-26 Waking and sleeping periods established. The baby is covered in vernix, a white, greasy substance that nourishes, protects and waterproofs the skin.

WEEK 27 The baby is starting to put on weight as it begins another growth spurt. The amount of amniotic fluid increases.

Nutrition for Mother & Baby

BY THE SECOND TRIMESTER, the nausea and extreme exhaustion of early pregnancy should be easing off. You will find that your energy levels increase and your appetite improves. Diet continues to be of great importance and certain nutrients are especially valuable at this stage of the baby's development.

FUELLING DEVELOPMENT

During the second trimester you will gain weight at the rate of about 450 g (1 lb) a week and your blood volume will increase. Progesterone will cause you to lay down fat to ensure there is enough "fuel" for milk production after the birth. The baby's development continues apace (*see page 47*). By the end of 14 weeks, its limbs are fully formed. By 21 weeks, the baby also will be laying down fat stores. Its nervous system is becoming more sophisticated and brain cells are multiplying at a staggering rate of at least 50,000 and 100,000 every minute. By the end of 24 weeks, the baby's other vital organs are maturing and the developing skeletal system is continuing to ossify.

KEY NUTRIENTS

Calcium is needed to form strong bones and teeth, to support muscle growth and to control nerve and muscle function in your baby. It is essential for you for blood clotting, and it may help to prevent raised blood pressure. Your need for calcium increases by a factor of at least three during pregnancy, although the ability of the body to absorb calcium becomes more efficient. Like calcium, phosphorus helps to form and maintain healthy bones and teeth. It is important for energy production and metabolism, and is needed for milk production. Magnesium is also essential for the baby's development, combining with calcium to build muscles, cells and nerves. It is needed for the functioning of the baby's liver and heart and for the metabolism of protein and carbohydrates.

KEY DAILY DIETARY CONSTITUENTS

7 servings of grains

6 servings of vegetables

4 servings of fruit, 2 of which are rich in vitamin C

3 servings of lean meat or pulses

3 servings of calcium-rich foods

3 servings of phosphorus-rich foods

3 servings of magnesium-rich foods

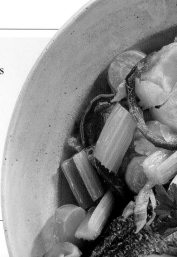

BAKED FISH WITH VEGETABLES *Fish such as grey mullet or bream, cooked with carrots, celery, peppers and garlic, supply protein and many nutrients.*

ESSENTIAL DIETARY NUTRIENTS

VITAMINS & MINERALS	FOR MOTHER	FOR BABY
VITAMIN A Half your intake of beta carotene may be converted into vitamin A.	*For maintaining immune system, healthy mucous membranes, bones, teeth, skin and hair.*	*For healthy neurons in the brain, cell membranes and vision.*
B VITAMINS Increased amounts are produced naturally in the body during pregnancy.	*B_6 and B_{12} to assist protein metabolism (extra protein is needed throughout pregnancy).*	*For development of nervous system, processing fatty acids and for energy.*
VITAMIN C This cannot be stored so regular intakes are necessary, but do not exceed 500 mg a day.	*For hormone production, boosting the immune system and iron absorption.*	*For collagen production, tissue growth, and healthy bones, teeth and skin.*
VITAMIN D The need for vitamin D increases throughout pregnancy, especially if not much time is spent outdoors.	*To store vitamin D to supply baby; for hormonal action and calcium and phosphate absorption.*	*For development of strong bones, especially foetal skull, and teeth.*
FOLATE The body stores very little folate so folic acid supplements will probably be needed.	*For hormonal action, protein metabolism, energy release, healthy nervous system.*	*For development of the nervous system, especially the spine.*
IRON The number of red blood cells in the body increases by 30 per cent during pregnancy.	*For haemoglobin production and prevention of anaemia.*	*For haemoglobin production.*
CALCIUM	*See* Key Nutrients, *opposite.*	*See* Key Nutrients, *opposite.*
PHOSPHORUS	*See* Key Nutrients, *opposite.*	*See* Key Nutrients, *opposite.*
MAGNESIUM	*See* Key Nutrients, *opposite.*	*See* Key Nutrients, *opposite.*

SECOND TRIMESTER

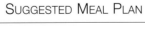

SUGGESTED MEAL PLAN

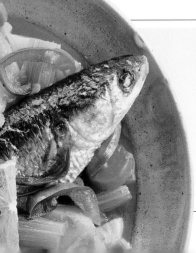

BREAKFAST
Cornflakes with sunflower seeds, banana and milk; wholemeal toast; orange juice

MIDMORNING SNACK
Walnuts and prunes

LUNCH
Wholemeal sandwich with salmon and avocado filling; kiwi fruit and a slice of melon

AFTERNOON SNACK
Houmous with carrot sticks

DINNER
Chicken stir-fry with beansprouts, ginger, baby corn, sesame seeds, mangetouts and brown rice

BEDTIME SNACK
Homemade popcorn

Exercise Plan

As far as exercise is concerned, the second trimester is about building up stamina and stretching your muscles. As your shape changes, you need to maintain good posture and target certain muscle groups to enable you to cope with the increasing physiological demands of pregnancy.

SECOND TRIMESTER

Key Tips

Stop exercising if you experience serious discomfort or pain

✳

Always correct your posture

✳

Do pelvic floor exercises daily

✳

Do not over-exert yourself

General Guidelines

You should at all times be aware of general guidelines relating to exercise during pregnancy (*see pages 18–19*). It is especially important to warm up before doing any form of exercise and to cool down when you have finished (*see page 32*).

Pelvic Exercises

Exercises for the pelvic area become increasingly important through pregnancy, and pelvic floor exercises should become part of your daily routine for the rest of your life.

• **Pelvic tilts** Stand with the feet hip-width apart and knees soft. Place one hand on the abdomen and the other on the bottom. Contract the abdominal muscles, tucking the bottom in and tilting the pelvis upwards. Alternatively, do pelvic tilts on all fours (*see opposite above*).

• **Pelvic floor exercises** These can be done at any stage of pregnancy (*see page 75*) and are also important after the birth.

Exercises for the Back

Dynamic changes are taking place within the pelvis at this time and a lot of pressure is being put on the spine because of the extra weight load at the front. Exercises to strengthen the back are therefore very important (*see page 33*).

Abdominal Exercises

Women are often nervous about doing abdominal exercises while pregnant, but are equally concerned about losing their shape and muscle tone, and especially in the stomach. From week 16 you should not do abdominal curls, but pelvic tilts (static abdominal contractions) are perfectly safe.

• **Abdominal curls** Stand in the same position as for pelvic tilts (*see above*). Place your hands

Correcting Posture

Standing up Straight
Stand with a straight back, shoulders back, and bottom tucked in to avoid putting strain on the back. Also, keep your back straight and supported when sitting down, with your feet flat on the floor.

Awareness of Position
Be aware of your body whatever you do. Kneel down rather than bending over; get up from lying down in easy stages; and bend the knees and keep the back straight when lifting.

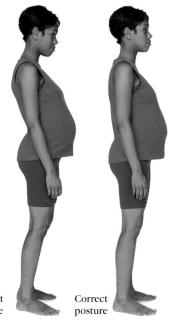

Incorrect posture

Correct posture

EXERCISES FOR PELVIS & STOMACH

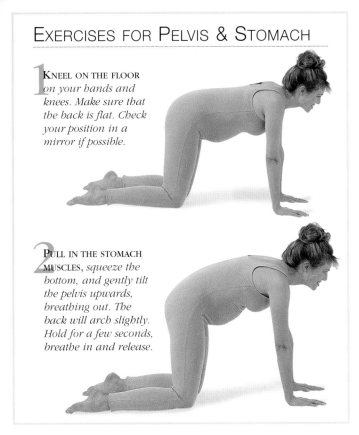

1 KNEEL ON THE FLOOR *on your hands and knees. Make sure that the back is flat. Check your position in a mirror if possible.*

2 PULL IN THE STOMACH MUSCLES, *squeeze the bottom, and gently tilt the pelvis upwards, breathing out. The back will arch slightly. Hold for a few seconds, breathe in and release.*

on your abdomen to either side of the baby. Breathe in deeply, then exhale, tucking your bottom in, tilting the pelvis upwards and contracting the abdominal muscles around the baby. Hold for a few seconds, then release, taking care not to arch the back.

PREVENTATIVE EXERCISES

As part of the muscle-strengthening section of your exercise programme (*see page 33*) you can include exercises that may help to prevent a

LEG CIRCLING
Lift the foot and flex it outwards. Draw large circles in the air. Repeat with the other foot.

variety of problems common to pregnancy. Many prevent or relieve aches and pains but other discomforts, such as cramp, heartburn and other forms of indigestion, can also be relieved by simple exercises.

IMPROVING CIRCULATION

Walking, swimming and gentle aerobic exercise (*see page 33*) are good for improving blood circulation. You can also try the following exercises.

• **Foot points and flexes** Sit with your back against a wedge

pillow or with your arms supporting you and your legs straight out in front. Point your toes and release about ten times. Then, pull your toes towards you, pressing the knees down and stretching the back of the calf. Hold for four seconds, breathing normally, then relax. Repeat five times.

• **Ankle circling** Keeping the hips still, circle each ankle, first one way, then the other. Also try leg circling (*see below*).

IMPROVING DIGESTION

To help prevent indigestion, bend down using your knees rather than from your waist, and lift things in the same way. The following simple yoga exercise might also help.

• **Relieving heartburn** To create more space below the diaphragm, sit with a straight back and palms together at chest level. Breathing in, lift the hands above your head; breathing out, lower the hands. Repeat several times.

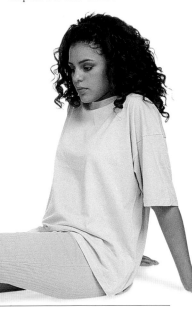

SECOND TRIMESTER

Five-point Action Plan

THIS IS THE TIME of the traditional "bloom" of pregnancy, and is for many women the most enjoyable stage. Sickness and exhaustion should be diminishing and, as you are more aware of the baby's movements, your confidence in the pregnancy should grow. You may "glow", and your appetite and energy should return. Bear in mind the following advice.

GO PUBLIC

You will start to notice the development of a "bump", and before too long your pregnancy will become obvious to other people, even if you have not yet told them about it. Now is the time to choose your antenatal classes and book them.

STAY FIT

As your energy returns, you may feel like exercising again. Be guided by your body and do not push yourself too hard. Enrol in exercise classes that are specially designed for pregnant women, such as aquanatal or yoga. As your shape changes and your ligaments relax, avoid jerky exercise movements or too much bending and lifting. Gentle stretching is preferable to strenuous aerobic exercise.

BUILD BODY SYSTEMS

Calcium and magnesium are used in the creation of strong bones and teeth in your baby and in the development of its muscles and nervous system. Make a point of eating foods that are rich in these minerals, such as sesame seeds, soya, almonds, dairy products and fish (for calcium) and oats, wheatgerm, rice and cabbage (for magnesium).

EAT THE RIGHT FOODS

It is not more food that you need, but more vitamins and minerals. Your baby takes what it needs from you, so it is important to replenish your own stocks of vital nutrients. As your blood volume increases, you need extra iron to prevent anaemia. Eat both iron-rich foods and sources of vitamin C, which assist iron absorption. You also need to eat plenty of fibre to prevent constipation.

LISTEN WITH MOTHER

Research suggests that from about week 20 of pregnancy your baby can hear and respond to sounds. Playing music to your baby may stimulate its brain cell activity and also provides you with an opportunity to put your feet up, relax and bond with your unborn child.

Common Problems
in the
Second
Trimester

EVEN THOUGH YOU ARE FEELING BETTER and you are more comfortable about your pregnancy, you may be affected by the common problems that tend to occur during the second trimester. The following natural solutions will enable to you to deal with them.

Heartburn

UP TO 80 PER CENT of pregnant women suffer from heartburn, a burning feeling in the chest and throat. Greater elasticity of the abdominal muscles can cause the valve at the entrance of the stomach to remain slightly open instead of closing tightly, so that stomach fluids return up the oesophagus. Heartburn tends to worsen as pregnancy progresses.

SYMPTOMS

*Sensation of burning
acid in the throat*

✳

Nausea

✳

*Unpleasant taste
in the mouth*

TRADITIONAL CHINESE BELIEFS

According to Traditional Chinese Medicine, the Stomach should be rested between 7 pm and 9 pm. To avoid heartburn, it is advisable for pregnant women to relax during this period and not eat. A light evening meal at about 6 pm and then a small snack before going to bed are preferable to a heavy evening meal. Eating light meals at the end of the day will enable you to sleep better.

✳ Reflexology may also help to alleviate heartburn. A practitioner will stimulate reflex points on the foot that correspond to the stomach and intestines in order to relieve your discomfort.

See pages 132 and 140–1 for further information

EARLY EVENING REST
To prevent or alleviate indigestion, relax during what is believed to be the Stomach's natural resting time of day.

KEY TIPS

*Eat several small meals
a day rather than one
or two large ones*

✳

*Sleep with several pillows
to keep your upper body
slightly raised*

✳

Wear loose-fitting clothes

✳

*Avoid bending over
suddenly*

✳

*Limit fluid intake at
meal times*

CAUTION

Do not take over-the-counter remedies or antacids for longer than is recommended. If symptoms persist, see your doctor.

COMPLEMENTARY TREATMENTS

Before using a treatment, please read any **Cautions** and the relevant page references

ACUPUNCTURE

In Traditional Chinese Medicine, heartburn is linked to excessive "heat" in the Stomach. An acupuncturist will seek to achieve balance in your digestive system, and will examine your tongue during diagnosis. The tip of the tongue represents the Heart, and is often red in women suffering from heartburn. The

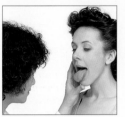

CHECKING THE TONGUE
The colour of the tongue is studied for clues about digestive ailments.

middle area of the tongue, representing the Stomach, may also be very red. The acupuncturist will attempt to clear excessive "heat" by treating specific acupoints, usually located on your arms or feet.

See pages 134–5 for further information

ACUPRESSURE

You can treat the appropriate acupuncture point yourself to relieve heartburn. Place four fingers at the point midway between the umbilicus (belly button) and the bottom of the breast bone. Press for ten seconds at a time over a period of 5–10 minutes.

See page 136 for further information

HOMEOPATHY

There are several homeopathic remedies for heartburn. A practitioner will select the appropriate one for you, based on a detailed description of your physical symptoms.

✱ For flatulence and discomfort in the digestive tract after eating, *Carbo veg. 6c.*

✱ For a heavy, full feeling in the stomach, *Nux vomica 6c.*

✱ For a gurgling, rumbling stomach, *Pulsatilla 6c.*

Caution: homeopathic remedies are neutralized by peppermint, a herbal remedy for heartburn.

See pages 148–9 for dosage and further information

WESTERN HERBALISM

Seeds such as caraway, dill and fennel may alleviate heartburn. They can be ground and added to food, or chewed whole after a meal. Also try the following self-help remedies:

✱ Drink soothing lemon balm, chamomile or peppermint teas throughout the day.

✱ Take slippery elm powder to ease flatulence: prepare by adding 5 g (1 tsp) each of slippery elm and honey to a cup of hot water.

See pages 150–1 for further information

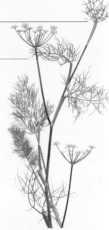

FENNEL PLANT
Seeds of the fennel plant, chewed or infused, make a palatable remedy.

AROMATHERAPY

For a soothing effect, massage the abdomen with four drops of an essential oil such as lavender added to a carrier oil. Use circular, clockwise movements for up to half an hour.

Caution: see page 153 for oils to avoid in pregnancy.

See pages 152–3 for further information

DIET & NUTRITION

Heartburn is aggravated by eating large meals and by certain combinations of foods. Some diets, such as the Hay Diet (*below*), are based on the premise that foods classed as acidic (such as proteins) should never be part of the same meal as alkaline foods (carbohydrates).

See pages 48–9 for further information

NEUTRAL FOODS
Some foods can be eaten freely with any others.

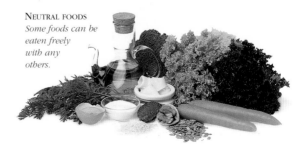

SECOND TRIMESTER

Anaemia

MANY PREGNANT WOMEN, particularly those expecting more than one baby, are anaemic. Anaemia occurs if the level of oxygen-carrying haemoglobin in red blood cells falls below normal. It is important to have healthy blood during pregnancy in order to prevent complications in labour due to fatigue, and to reduce susceptibility to postnatal depression.

SYMPTOMS

Dizziness, palpitations, pale skin

✳

Lethargy, general malaise, emotional fragility

✳

Constipation may be a side effect of taking iron

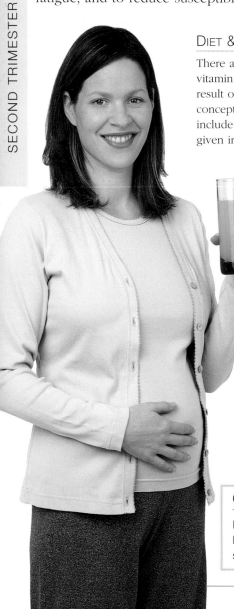

DIET & NUTRITION

There are three main causes of anaemia: deficiency in iron, folate or vitamin B^{12}. Iron deficiency is the most common in pregnancy as a result of demand from the baby. Women with heavy periods before conception may enter pregnancy slightly anaemic. Antenatal checks include blood tests. If you are diagnosed as anaemic, you will be given iron tablets. Anaemia can occur even if you have an iron-rich diet, since it may be due to a lack of B vitamins. The following dietary guidelines will help to remedy anaemia: the nutrients listed cannot be stored in the body so eat good food sources every day.

✳ To prevent iron deficiency, eat plenty of green leafy vegetables, pumpkin seeds, cherries, dried apricots, fish and poultry. Drink blackcurrant and cranberry juices.

✳ To remedy vitamin B^{12} deficiency, eat eggs, milk, cheese, white fish, pork and yeast extract.

✳ To reduce folate deficiency, eat nuts and raw or steamed green leafy vegetables, wheatgerm, yeast extract and pulses.

See pages 48–9 for further information

IMPROVING IRON ABSORPTION
Consuming vitamin C – such as in fresh orange juice – with iron-rich foods improves absorption of the mineral.

KEY TIPS

Eat vitamin C-rich foods with iron-rich ones

✳

Avoid too many calcium-rich foods, which inhibit iron absorption

CAUTION

If you suspect that you are anaemic, see your doctor. Anaemia lowers resistance to infection and may cause muscle contractions since the blood is carrying insufficient oxygen.

COMPLEMENTARY TREATMENTS

Before using a complementary treatment, please read any **Cautions** and the relevant page references

ACUPUNCTURE

Traditional Chinese Medicine considers the Blood to be responsible for both physical and emotional well-being. If a person's Blood volume is low, their spirits may also be low, which might explain why pregnant women are often tearful or depressed if they are anaemic. To diagnose anaemia, a practitioner will look at your tongue, which may be pale and dry. You will also be asked to describe your symptoms. Anxiety, palpitations, dream-disturbed sleep or sleeplessness may all be of significance in TCM diagnosis. An acupuncturist commonly addresses the blood points in the treatment of anaemia.

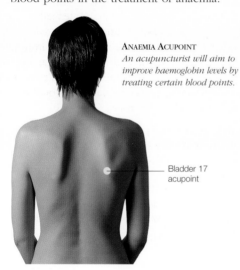

ANAEMIA ACUPOINT
An acupuncturist will aim to improve haemoglobin levels by treating certain blood points.

Bladder 17 acupoint

✳ There are certain points along the meridians that an acupuncturist will treat in order to build up the blood. If you are feeling particularly weak and tired, these points may be heated first with moxa cones.

See pages 134–5 for further information

ACUPRESSURE

Acupressure – which is acupuncture without needles – is based on the same principles of stimulating points along the body's meridians through which life energy flows. It is particularly suitable for self-help application

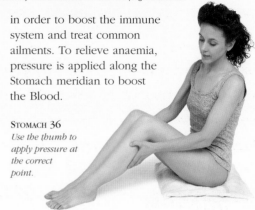

in order to boost the immune system and treat common ailments. To relieve anaemia, pressure is applied along the Stomach meridian to boost the Blood.

STOMACH 36
Use the thumb to apply pressure at the correct point.

✳ Sit on the floor with your knees bent. Place each thumb just beyond the knee bones, where you feel a depression. Press for three seconds four or five times and do this two or three times a day.

See page 136 for further information

HOMEOPATHY

Ferrum phos. and *Calc. phos.* tissue salts can be taken by women with iron-deficiency anaemia as a self-help measure to improve the absorption of iron. Those with other types of anaemia should consult a homeopath, who will prescribe constitutionally, for example:

✳ For pale lips and physical and mental exhaustion, *Ferrum met. 6c.*

See pages 148–9 for dosage and further information

WESTERN HERBALISM

Nettle tea is a tonic and a rich source of minerals, including iron. Steep 5 g (1 tsp) of the dried herb in a cup of freshly boiled water for 10–15 minutes. Drink 1–4 cups a day.

See pages 150–1 for further information

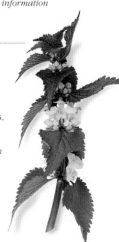

NETTLE
High in both vitamin C and iron, nettle makes a good tonic for women with anaemia.

Backache, Symphysis Pubic Pain & Sciatica

SECOND TRIMESTER

BACKACHE IN PREGNANCY OFTEN OCCURS as a result of ligaments and joints being softened by hormonal action. In the pelvis, this leads to symphysis pubic pain, which makes it difficult to sleep or do chores such as shopping. Sciatica may be caused by pressure exerted on nerves by the baby, causing numbness or weakness in the buttocks, thighs and legs.

SYMPTOMS

Pain along the spine or in the pelvis
*

Weakness or pain in the buttocks and legs
*

Walking hampered by pain in the feet or legs

OSTEOPATHY

Changes in posture can be a source of strain, and the baby's position can exacerbate **backache**, especially if the baby is lying with its back facing the mother's spine. Pelvic joints can be the worst affected by hormones: the joints soften in order to stretch during labour. This puts pressure on the spine and pelvis and often causes **symphysis pubic pain**. Osteopathy can help to ease the strain on the musculo-skeletal system caused by pregnancy. An osteopath may manipulate the sacroiliac joints by rotating the pelvis slightly, so relieving pressure on the ligaments.

✳ To support the back and relieve pain, you may be advised to wear a fembrace. This is a belt that slips around the back and under the baby, helping to support the back.

See page 146 for further information

KEY TIPS

Listen to your body and avoid doing things that cause discomfort
*

Rest and take the weight off the pelvis whenever possible
*

Swimming is good exercise for back problems
*

Wear some sort of pelvic support

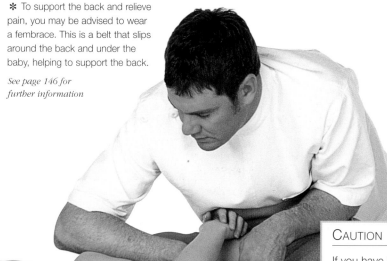

EASING BACK PAIN
An osteopath will examine each vertebra to detect and correct any restriction in its range of movement.

CAUTION

If you have backache accompanied by abdominal pain before 36 weeks, contact your doctor since you might be going into premature labour.

COMPLEMENTARY TREATMENTS

Before using a complementary treatment, please read any **Cautions** and the relevant page references

ACUPUNCTURE

After studying your medical history, a practitioner will investigate the degree and location of **backache**, and whether or not it is affected by heat or cold. Fine needles will be inserted into the back and legs, or into the pubic bone to relieve **symphysis pubic pain**.

✳ According to Traditional Chinese Medicine, the bones are governed by the Kidney meridian. The peak time for this meridian is from 5 pm to 7 pm, so try to rest during this period to get maximum benefit.

✳ In the last month of pregnancy, a TENS machine (*see page 109*) can be of benefit to the lower back.

Caution: do not use a TENS machine before 36 weeks since as it can stimulate uterine contractions.

See pages 134–5 for further information

REFLEXOLOGY

A reflexologist will gently massage the inner edges of your feet, which may provide temporary relief for **backache**.

See pages 140–1 for further information

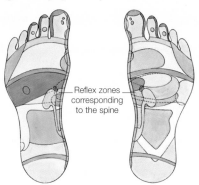

Reflex zones corresponding to the spine

REFLEXOLOGY
Working along a line down the inner edge of each foot may ease spine-related ailments.

YOGA

Some yoga positions can help to relieve **backache**. Sitting on your heels, lower your body forwards, putting your hands on the floor and keeping your back straight. Leaning on your elbows, lower yourself further so that you are resting your head on your arms on

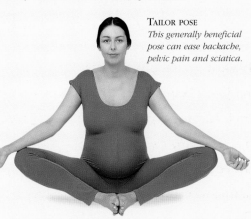

TAILOR POSE
This generally beneficial pose can ease backache, pelvic pain and sciatica.

the floor. Your bump should rest comfortably between your knees, supported by the floor. Alternatively, try the tailor pose (*see above*).

See page 142 for further information

CHIROPRACTIC

Backache, **symphysis pubic pain** and **sciatica** may all be eased by chiropractic. A practitioner will realign vertebrae in the lower back, and relieve torsion (twisting), thus soothing irritated spinal nerves.

See page 147 for further information

ALEXANDER TECHNIQUE

As pregnancy progresses, your centre of gravity shifts with your changing body shape. An Alexander teacher can teach you to be more aware of the way you move and carry yourself.

See page 147 for further information

MASSAGE

Backache can benefit from massage. Ask your partner to massage your back along either side of the spine, using an essential oil in a carrier oil such as almond.

See pages 152–3 for further information

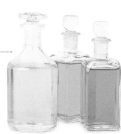

CARRIER OILS
These oils are used to dilute essential oils for use in massage.

SECOND TRIMESTER

Migraine & Headaches

TEN PER CENT OF PREGNANT WOMEN suffer from migraine – a severe headache caused by the dilation of blood vessels in the brain and linked to the hormonal changes that occur in pregnancy. Headaches also can be caused by hormonal action, or by stress or tension in the muscles of the head and neck as a result of poor posture during pregnancy.

SYMPTOMS

Dull thudding in the head, worse for moving

❋

Pain on one side of the head or in the temples

❋

Numbness, vomiting or visual disturbances

ACUPRESSURE

According to Traditional Chinese Medicine, headaches in early pregnancy are often caused by blockages of the Liver and the Gall Bladder meridians, preventing the flow of *qi*, or life energy. To relieve headaches by improving the flow of *qi*, stimulate acupoints on the head.

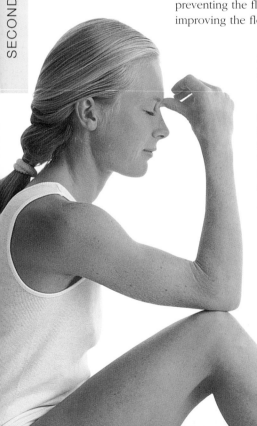

❋ A headache may be relieved by stimulating the acupoints Gallbladder 20 at the back of the neck and the base of the skull.

❋ A migraine may be eased by applying pressure to the *yintang* point between the eyebrows, just above the bridge of your nose, with your thumb. Massage this point of pain, using a gentle, circular movement.

See page 136 for further information

SOOTHING PRESSURE
To relax and therefore help to ease a migraine, close your eyes and press gently between your eyebrows with your thumb.

KEY TIPS

Get plenty of fresh air each day

❋

Take 20 minutes' gentle exercise each day

❋

Sleep and rest as much as possible

❋

Drink plenty of filtered or mineral water

❋

Try to reduce your stress levels

CAUTIONS

Consult your doctor before continuing to take drugs prescribed for migraine before you were pregnant. Report persistent headaches after 24 weeks to your midwife or doctor, since they may be indicative of other conditions.

COMPLEMENTARY TREATMENTS

Before using a complementary treatment, please read any **Cautions** and the relevant page references

ACUPUNCTURE

According to the Chinese, climatic factors such as damp cause headaches. Precise symptoms are important: pain centred on the temples, for example, indicates Gall Bladder imbalance, and a practitioner will treat points on the relevant meridian at the back of the neck.

See pages 134–5 for further information

REIKI

Reiki energy is believed to flow to where it is needed in the body. The treatment is relaxing, helping to ease a stress-related headache.

See page 139 for further information

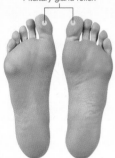

Pituitary gland reflex

REFLEXOLOGY

The big toes will be stimulated by a reflexologist to help to relieve a migraine.

See pages 140–1 for further information

RELIEVING MIGRAINE
The tip of the big toe is the pituitary gland reflex zone, which is stimulated in the treatment of migraine.

CHIROPRACTIC

Recurrent headaches or migraines may be due to a misalignment of the vertebrae, putting pressure on the nerves. A chiropractor will manipulate the area to correct this.

See page 147 for further information

HOMEOPATHY

Depending on your specific symptoms, one of the following remedies may be prescribed:

✳ For sudden pain resembling a tight band, *Aconite 6c*.

✳ For sudden, violent headache, *Belladonna 6c*.

✳ For irritability and pain that is worse for movement and that lasts all day, *Bryonia 6c*.

See pages 148–9 for dosage and further information

WESTERN HERBALISM

Chamomile tea is soothing if you have a headache; ginger tea acts as a circulatory tonic.

See pages 150–1 for further information

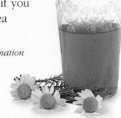

CHAMOMILE TEA
Calming chamomile tea makes an effective headache remedy.

AROMATHERAPY

Four drops of lavender oil, applied on a compress to the temples, relieves a headache.

Caution: see page 153 for oils to avoid in pregnancy.

See pages 152–3 for further information

MASSAGE

A relaxing neck and shoulder massage can relieve a headache by easing muscle tension and improving blood circulation.

See pages 152–3 for further information

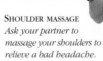

SHOULDER MASSAGE
Ask your partner to massage your shoulders to relieve a bad headache.

DIET & NUTRITION

Headaches are commonly caused during pregnancy by dehydration or low blood sugar levels. Drink plenty of water and follow these dietary guidelines:

✳ Stabilize blood sugar levels by eating slow-release carbohydrates (porridge, bread, pulses, starchy root vegetables and wholegrains) and protein regularly.

✳ Avoid eating migraine-causing foods including chocolate, caffeine, alcohol, citrus fruit and cheese.

See pages 48–9 for further information

SECOND TRIMESTER

Constipation, Haemorrhoids & Varicose Veins

SECOND TRIMESTER

CONSTIPATION IS COMMON in pregnancy because the hormone progesterone slows bowel movements. Constipation or pressure from the uterus may lead to swollen veins, or haemorrhoids, in the lining of the anus. Pressure on the circulatory system, due to increased weight and blood volume, may enlarge and distort veins, especially in the legs.

SYMPTOMS

Infrequent or difficult passage of faeces

❋

Protruding, painful possibly bleeding veins in the anus

❋

Large, raised veins on legs

ACUPUNCTURE

In Traditional Chinese Medicine, the back of the tongue represents the bowels, and a practitioner will examine this area to see if there is a yellow coating, which indicates constipation. If so, "heat" acupoints, which lie along the Large Intestine meridian, may be stimulated. A practitioner might also treat the following points:

❋ Relieve the pain from **haemorrhoids** by stimulating the Bladder meridian on the back of the calf. Another good acupoint lies on the top of the head.

❋ Ease the pain of knotted **varicose veins**, by inserting needles superficially around the troublesome vein itself.

See pages 134–5 for further information

KEY TIPS

To ease constipation, go on long walks, drink lots of water and eat foods that are high in fibre

❋

To relieve haemorrhoids get lots of rest, do gentle exercise, drink plenty of water and avoid tea, coffee and spicy foods

❋

Alleviate varicose veins by taking daily exercise and wearing support tights

EASING HAEMORRHOIDS
Fine acupuncture needles may be inserted into your head for the relief of haemorrhoids.

CAUTION

If you feel a deep, niggling pain in your calf, or if there is a feeling of heaviness in that area, contact your doctor immediately, as this may be indicative of deep-vein thrombosis.

COMPLEMENTARY TREATMENTS

Before using a complementary treatment, please read any **Cautions** and the relevant page references

ACUPRESSURE

Constipation can be helped by stimulating the acupoint halfway along a line from the pubic bone to the belly button. Apply finger pressure intermittently for ten seconds.

See page 136 for further information

YOGA

To help ease **haemorrhoids** or **varicose veins**, try holding gentle, inverted yoga postures. A simple, beneficial position is to lie with the feet and legs raised against a wall for 15–30 minutes twice a day.

See page 142 for further information

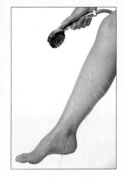

HOT AND COLD SHOWER
Hot followed by cold water can ease the discomfort of varicose veins.

HYDROTHERAPY

To reduce **varicose veins** temporarily, place your leg (up to the calf) in hot water for two minutes, then cold water for two minutes. Alternatively, direct a shower spray on to the affected area, first with hot water, then with cold.

See page 144 for further information

HOMEOPATHY

One of the following self-help remedies may be beneficial in combating **haemorrhoids**, depending on your particular symptoms:

✱ For internal haemorrhoids that bleed, are very painful and are better for bathing in warm water, *Arsen. alb. 6c*.

✱ For bleeding, protruding haemorrhoids that itch and are better for bathing in cold water, *Nux vomica 6c*.

✱ For large, sore, bleeding haemorrhoids that occur towards the end of pregnancy, *Hamamelis 6c*.

✱ For oozing, painful, protruding haemorrhoids, *Sepia 6c*.

See pages 148–9 for dosage and further information

DANDELION
Roots of the dandelion plant may improve bowel function.

WESTERN HERBALISM

To relieve **constipation**, drink hot water with lemon or dandelion root decoction before breakfast. Apply the following herbal remedies to help to ease **haemorrhoids**: St. John's wort ointment that has been kept in a refrigerator; cold witch hazel or nettle tea compresses; grated raw potato or carrot (put directly on the affected area); or ice cubes, made from water in which leeks were boiled. **Varicose veins** may be eased by applying commercially available preparations of calendula or aloe vera or witch hazel compresses.

See pages 150–1 for further information

AROMATHERAPY

Abdominal massage may help **constipation**. Use any essential oil that you find pleasant
Caution: see page 153 for oils to avoid in pregnancy.
See pages 152–3 for further information

DIET & NUTRITION

To remedy **haemorrhoids** or **varicose veins**, or to prevent them, eat vein-strengthening foods that are rich in vitamin C and bioflavonoids, such as parsley, garlic and onions. The following will help constipation:

✱ Drink lots of water.

✱ Limit processed foods and eat plenty of fibre.

✱ Eat psyllium seeds and linseed to soften the stools.

✱ Eat oat bran, dried fruits, cabbage, peas, papayas and figs.

✱ Eat almonds and bananas for bulk and honey for lubrication.

See pages 48–9 for further information

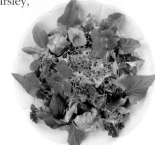

SALAD BOWL
Two or three helpings of salad a day will provide plenty of useful fibre.

SECOND TRIMESTER

Cystitis, Thrush & Herpes

CYSTITIS IS COMMON in pregnancy, and is caused by bacteria that inflame the lining of the bladder. Thrush, a vaginal infection, also often affects pregnant women. The *herpes simplex* virus can cause cold sores and genital herpes. Women with genital herpes may require a Caesarean section if symptoms flare up before or during labour.

SYMPTOMS

Pain and frequent urge to pass urine (cystitis)

✳

Itching and white discharge (thrush)

✳

Flu-like symptoms preceding sores (herpes)

AROMATHERAPY

Essential oils that benefit the urinary tract include chamomile, geranium and lavender. Four drops of oil can be added to a bath or put on a warm compress over the pubic bone or the kidneys. Relaxing oils ease stress, thus helping to keep the herpes virus dormant.

✳ Add 3–4 drops of uplifting lemon balm oil to a bath or place a few drops in a vaporizer for pain relief.

✳ Place a chamomile compress over the kidneys to remedy **thrush** or add 3–4 drops of tea tree oil to a bowl of warm water and use as an antiseptic douche.

Caution: see page 153 for oils to avoid in pregnancy.

See pages 152–3 for further information

KEY TIPS

To ease cystitis, drink about 2.5 litres (4½ pints) of water a day. Pour warm water over the entrance to the urethra while sitting on the toilet

✳

Eat plenty of fresh fruit and vegetables to guard against thrush and herpes

✳

Help prevent herpes from flaring up by resting and avoiding stress

RELAXING OILS
Essential oils such as lavender or chamomile, added to your bath water, may ease stress, helping the body to resist infection.

CAUTIONS

Avoid sexual intercourse if you have cystitis. Herpes is highly infectious: do not have sexual intercourse if you believe that an outbreak is about to occur. If you have backache and a temperature, consult your doctor since you may have a urinary tract infection, which may trigger premature labour.

COMPLEMENTARY TREATMENTS

Before using a complementary treatment, please read any **Cautions** and the relevant page references

REFLEXOLOGY

Symptoms of **cystitis** may be relieved by reflex zone therapy. A reflexologist will stimulate the kidney and other urinary reflex points on the feet in an attempt to disperse the toxins that are responsible for the inflammation of the urinary system. It is advisable to consult a qualified reflexologist who has had previous experience of treating pregnant women.

See pages 140–1 for further information

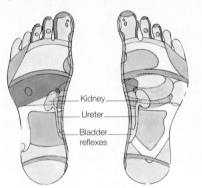

Kidney
Ureter
Bladder
reflexes

TREATING CYSTITIS
A reflexologist will work down each foot from kidney to bladder zones.

HYDROTHERAPY

To treat **thrush**, clean the affected area in a shower or bidet. Add 15–30 ml (1–2 tbsp) cider apple vinegar to warm water and douche: this may sting. Apply live yogurt for two hours.

See page 144 for further information

HOMEOPATHY

Self-help remedies can be taken alongside antibiotics for urinary tract infections.

✳ For **cystitis** with a burning sensation along the ureter and bright red, bloody urine, *Belladonna 6c.*
✳ For **herpes** with an itchy, stinging rash, *Capsicum 6c.*
✳ For **herpes** with skin that is red and dry and lesions that are hot and puffy with blisters, *Natrum mur. 6c.*

See page 148–9 for dosage and further information

WESTERN HERBALISM

Calendula ointment can soothe **thrush**, as can antifungal lavender or tea tree pessaries. To ease **herpes**, dab the affected area with calendula oil, St John's wort oil or aloe vera gel. Also try the following:

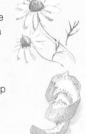

✳ Nettle or dandelion tea acts as a diuretic to flush out **cystitis**.
✳ Five drops each of St John's wort and calendula tinctures added to 1 litre (1¾ pints) cooled water and used as a douche three times a day and before bed, to relieve **thrush**.
✳ One or two cups a day of either chamomile or lemon balm tea may help to keep the **herpes** virus dormant.

See pages 150–1 for further information

DIET & NUTRITION

Drink plenty of water to flush out the urinary system and ease **cystitis**. Cranberry juice will also help to alleviate symptoms. To help prevent **herpes**, eat plenty of garlic, fresh fruit and lysine-rich foods such as fresh fish, chicken, beef, milk, cheese, eggs, beans and fresh vegetables. A daily 500 mg supplement of vitamin C will also be beneficial. Bear in mind the following dietary guidelines:

✳ A diet that includes beetroot, tomatoes and citrus fruit is likely to aggravate **cystitis.**
✳ Foods containing yeast and sugar should be avoided in order to prevent **thrush**.
✳ Foods that are rich in the amino acid arginine, such as nuts, seeds, wheat, brown rice and chocolate, as well as foods containing sugar, should be limited to help to prevent **herpes**.

See pages 48–9 for further information

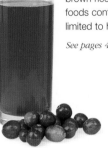

CRANBERRIES
These are believed to prevent cystitis bacteria from sticking to the bladder wall.

SECOND TRIMESTER

Depression

DEPRESSION IN PREGNANCY can occur for simple or complex reasons. Hormonal changes affect both your emotional and physical state, and can cause nausea, exhaustion and mood swings. Having a baby involves changes to your personal circumstances – there is a loss of freedom, for example – and old, buried fears and concerns can surface at this time.

SYMPTOMS

Negative feelings, mood swings or detachment

❋

Disturbed sleep

❋

Panic attacks

❋

Changes in appetite

YOGA

Yoga can be particularly effective in the treatment of depression, whatever the underlying cause. There are many different forms of yoga but they all aim, by means of breathing techniques and postures, to balance mind and body, thus leading to physical relaxation and improved spiritual well-being.

❋ Alternate nostril breathing can help to relax you, which it turn relieves depression. Rest your first two fingers on the front of your forehead, just above your nose, which is the location of the *yintang* acupoint. Then, with your thumb blocking one nostril, breathe in to a count of four, then breathe out to a count of four. Next, release your thumb and cover your other nostril with your ring finger. Breathe in and out as before. Repeat this exercise for several minutes.

See page 142 for further information

ALTERNATE NOSTRIL BREATHING
Combined with acupressure, this deep-breathing technique is believed to calm the mind and lift depression.

KEY TIPS

Discuss your feelings with a counsellor or friend

❋

Avoid eating sugary or highly refined foods

❋

Avoid stimulants such as caffeinated drinks, cigarettes and alcohol

CAUTION

If you feel depressed, do not be reluctant to tell your doctor or midwife how you feel: do not suffer alone. Counselling can be as effective as anti-depressant drugs in relieving mild to moderate depression.

COMPLEMENTARY TREATMENTS

Before using a complementary treatment, please read any **Cautions** and the relevant page references

ACUPUNCTURE

Acupuncture is excellent for treating depression. It encourages the release of neurotransmitters in the brain that relieve depressive symptoms.

See pages 134–5 for further information

REIKI

Reiki can be effective in treating depression. Some people report that it helps on an emotional level, lifting the spirits and creating feelings of calm and well-being.

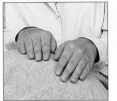

See page 139 for further information

REIKI
The practitioner's hands are believed to transmit healing energy.

HOMEOPATHY

If you have serious or chronic depression, consult a homeopathic practitioner for constitutional treatment. The following self-help remedies may bring relief for mild to moderate depression, however:

✴ For depression with wildly fluctuating mood swings, *Ignatia 30c*.

✴ For tearfulness that is worse for heat, *Pulsatilla 30c*.

✴ If you feel withdrawn and resentful, *Natrum mur. 30c*.

Caution: replace tea and coffee with herbal teas while you are taking homeopathic preparations.

See pages 148–9 for dosage and further information

WESTERN HERBALISM

St John's wort is an effective herbal remedy for treating nervous disorders and emotional upset. Taken internally as an infusion or a tincture, it is believed to relieve anxiety, nervous tension leading to exhaustion, irritability and mild depression.

Caution: consult your doctor before taking St John's wort if you are taking any conventional medication.

See pages 150–1 for further information

AROMATHERAPY

Certain essential oils can affect the nervous system and help to lift the spirits. Citrus oils, such as orange blossom, mandarin and grapefruit are particularly effective. You could also try lavender or rose oil. Use a couple of drops of oil, either added to a bath, in a vaporizer, or blended with a carrier oil for massage.

Caution: see page 153 for oils to avoid in pregnancy.

See pages 152–3 for further information

FLOWER REMEDIES

Gentle flower remedies may be effective for emotional problems. Take them individually or combine up to five remedies: put a few drops of each remedy in a 20 ml dropper bottle and top up with still mineral water.

✴ Elm eases a sense of overwhelming responsibilitiy.
✴ Gentian counteracts despondency and negativity.
✴ Holly eases anger and a feeling of lacking love.
✴ Mimulus calms those full of fear.
✴ Borage soothes depression caused by circumstances.

See page 154 for further information

DIET & NUTRITION

Nutritional deficiencies can cause hormonal imbalance, which affects emotional health. Zinc deficiency is common during pregnancy, so eat zinc-rich foods such as eggs, sunflower seeds and wholemeal bread. Also boost intake of vitamins C and B complex. Avoid sugary foods and stimulants such as caffeine and alcohol which can all adversely affect mood.

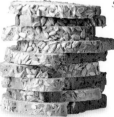

See pages 48–9 for further information

WHOLEMEAL BREAD
An excellent source of zinc and vitamin B⁶, wholemeal bread is a slow-release carbohydrate and will help to stabilize mood.

SECOND TRIMESTER

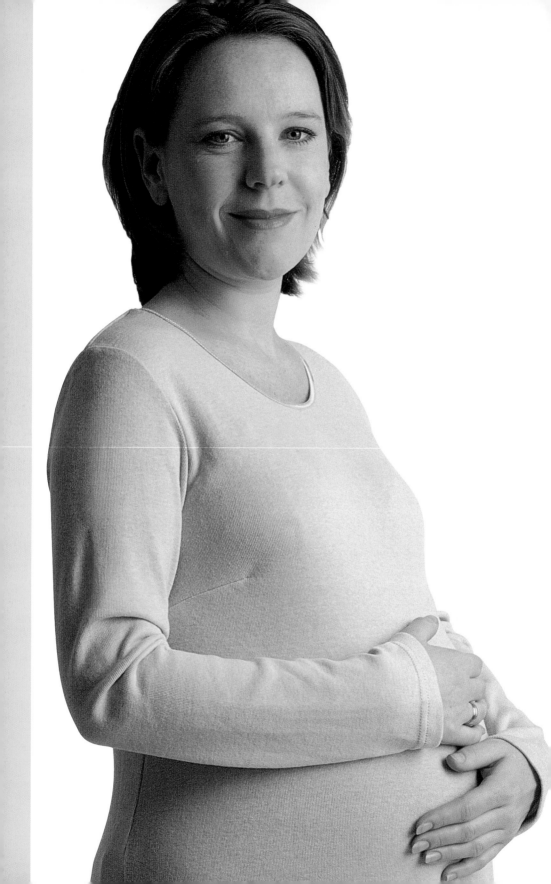

THE FINAL THREE MONTHS of pregnancy are an important time of preparation, when you need to gear yourself up nutritionally, emotionally and physically for the birth of your baby. Many women are still working, but the importance of getting sufficient rest cannot be over-emphasized. Blood volume is increasing by 40 per cent, pelvic joints

The third trimester

are expanding, breast tissue is developing and the baby is growing faster than at any other time during pregnancy. Plenty of rest can help to alleviate some of the ailments that occur in the third trimester as well as fortifying you for the birth. Complementary therapies, good nutrition and appropriate exercise can also help with this preparation.

Development of Mother & Baby

YOU MAY FEEL AS IF YOU HAVE BEEN PREGNANT for ever. At any time now you will start to produce colostrum and experience the first "practice" (Braxton Hicks) contractions, which are irregular and painless. Pelvic joints and ligaments are expanding ready for the birth.

THIRD TRIMESTER

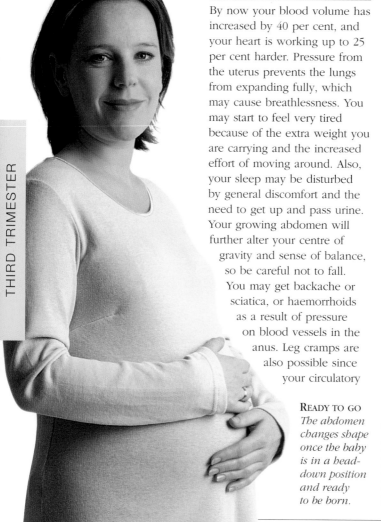

PHYSICAL DEVELOPMENTS

By now your blood volume has increased by 40 per cent, and your heart is working up to 25 per cent harder. Pressure from the uterus prevents the lungs from expanding fully, which may cause breathlessness. You may start to feel very tired because of the extra weight you are carrying and the increased effort of moving around. Also, your sleep may be disturbed by general discomfort and the need to get up and pass urine. Your growing abdomen will further alter your centre of gravity and sense of balance, so be careful not to fall. You may get backache or sciatica, or haemorrhoids as a result of pressure on blood vessels in the anus. Leg cramps are also possible since your circulatory

READY TO GO
The abdomen changes shape once the baby is in a head-down position and ready to be born.

system is working twice as hard as it usually does. By 32–33 weeks you will be gaining weight faster than at any other time in pregnancy. You will be feeling very heavy, having gained 8.5–11.25 kg (21–7 lb). Blood flow through the placenta has reached 450 litres (100 gal) a day. Overwork or lack of rest will impede this and affect the baby's growth.

READY FOR BIRTH

You should begin antenatal classes at about week 32. In 57 per cent of pregnancies the baby will turn after week 32 so that it is head-down; a further 25 per cent turn after week 36. At any time from then on the head will engage in the pelvis. Engagement is a preparation for labour but it does not mean that the birth is imminent. Some babies do not engage until after labour has begun. By week 37 weight gain will be slowing, although some women may suffer from water retention. By week 38 you will be feeling large and uncomfortable, and Braxton Hicks contractions may be strong and frequent.

THE BABY'S DEVELOPMENT

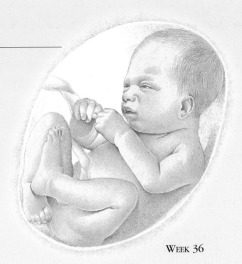

WEEK 28 Eyes are open sometimes and developing the ability to focus. If born now the baby would, with special care, have a good chance of survival. A boy's testes now descend into the groin.

WEEK 29 The baby is about 34 cm (13½ in) in length and covered with vernix. The lungs have developed most of their alveoli and are producing surfactant, a wetting agent, to assist breathing.

WEEK 30 During several weeks of moving around, the baby has increased muscle tone and developed the ability to orientate itself in space. Very occasionally it will turn so that it is in a head-down position.

WEEK 31 The skin is becoming pink rather than red as a result of the white fat deposits that have been laid down beneath it. These will provide energy and regulate temperature after the baby is born.

WEEK 32 The vernix is very thick and there may be quite a lot of hair on the head. Fingernails are fully grown but toenails are not. The face is smooth by now with few wrinkles.

WEEK 33 The baby is almost completely formed and in the proportions you would expect to see at birth. It is gaining weight. The body systems are still maturing.

WEEK 34 The brain and nervous system are fully developed. The immune system is still immature and the baby continues to receive its mother's antibodies. It is about 37 cm (15 in) in length.

WEEK 36

WEEK 35 The baby's movements may start to slow down now as there is less room to manoeuvre.

WEEK 36 Seventy per cent of the oxygen and nutrients coming through the placenta are used by the brain. If the baby were born now, it would be mature enough to survive without too many problems. More fat is accumulating under the skin. Meconium, a dark green, thick substance made up of dead cells and secretions from the bowel and liver, is being produced in the intestines.

WEEK 37 The baby will be practising breathing, sucking and swallowing. Its level of consciousness and degree of co-ordination will by this stage be well established.

WEEK 38 The baby is ready to be born. (Its development has taken 38 weeks from the moment of conception. Forty weeks of pregnancy is calculated from the first day of your last menstrual period.) The baby is plump and only just fits inside the uterus. It has to curl up tightly. The head will now descend into the lower part of the uterus and press through the softened, partially opened cervix, ready for the birth.

THIRD TRIMESTER

Nutrition for Mother & Baby

THERE ARE, AS IN THE FIRST TWO TRIMESTERS, windows of nutritional opportunity during the last three months of pregnancy. This period includes the time when you should be preparing your body for giving birth (*see also pages 98–9*), but also providing sustenance for crucial brain growth in your baby prior to the birth.

KEY TIPS

Make sure that the fats in your diet are mainly polyunsaturated

✳

Include plenty of foods rich in iron and vitamin C in your diet

✳

Eat plenty of "brain foods"

FUELLING DEVELOPMENT

Your blood volume is still increasing, so you need plenty of iron-rich foods as well as vitamin C for good absorption of the iron. You are gaining weight faster than at any other time in the pregnancy, laying down fat ready for producing milk. It is important to eat the right kind of fat – that is, polyunsaturated – to obtain essential fatty acids.

CRUCIAL BRAIN FOOD

The baby's brain is growing faster than ever. The number of brain cells is increasing at a rate of at least 100,000 a minute. Seventy per cent of the calories your baby receives are used for brain growth. When the baby is born, its brain weighs about 350 g (12 oz). Sixty per cent of it is made up of fat, and 20 per cent of that is composed of long-chain polyunsaturated fatty acids (LCPs). These "essential" fatty acids are required for the rapid transmission of signals between nerve cells. There are two kinds of essential fatty acids, both essential for good brain function: linoleic acid (omega–6) and linolenic acid (omega–3). The best food sources of omega–6 are seeds and their oils. The best sources of omega–3 are linseed, pumpkin seeds and oily fish. One of the active forms of omega–3 is DHA (docosahexaenoic acid), which is a component of brain-cell membranes and ensures good neural connections. There is evidence that DHA may help to prevent pregnancy-induced hypertension (raised blood pressure), and that it reduces the risk of premature birth, increases a baby's birth weight, improves its IQ and visual and cognitive brain function and also protects against heart disease.

KEY DAILY DIETARY CONSTITUENTS

7 servings of grains
6 servings of vegetables
4 servings of fruit, 2 of which are rich in vitamin C
3 servings of lean meat, fish or pulses
2 servings of calcium-rich food
1 serving of magnesium-rich food

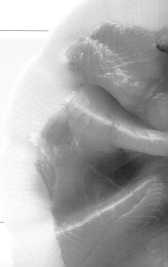

SMOKED SALMON SALAD
The fish provides valuable protein ready for labour and breastfeeding; the salad is light yet nutritious.

ESSENTIAL DIETARY NUTRIENTS

NUTRIENTS	FOR MOTHER	FOR BABY
VITAMIN A This is a powerful anti-oxidant.	*For production of hormones for lactation and good immunity.*	*For maintaining healthy mucous membranes.*
B VITAMINS Vitamins B2 is needed in increased amounts as well as those listed (*see* For Mother, *right*).	*B¹ for energy production; B⁶ for protein metabolism; folate to make DNA and (with B¹²) to make red blood cells.*	*B¹ for energy production.*
VITAMIN E This is a powerful anti-oxidant.	*Speeds up wound healing; increases skin suppleness; may strengthen uterine muscles.*	*For development of the nervous system and heart.*
OTHER VITAMINS K is made naturally in the gut, but not in a baby's, so it may be given orally at birth.	*C for iron absorption, hormone production, and resistance to infection; K for blood clotting.*	*K for blood clotting.*
CALCIUM Foetus takes up calcium at a rate of about 350 mg a day.	*For prevention of pre-eclampsia and raised blood pressure; (with vitamin D) to ease labour pains.*	*For development of bones and teeth.*
ZINC Boys take five times as much zinc as girls: deficiency is linked to undescended testes.	*For hormonal balance; may help to prevent stretch marks.*	*For development and growth of reproductive system.*
OTHER MINERALS Iron intake must be kept high because it takes six weeks to build up supplies.	*Iron for manufacture of red blood cells (vitamins C, B⁶, B¹² and folate improve absorpion).*	*Selenium for brain development; phosphorus for bone development.*

THIRD TRIMESTER

SUGGESTED MEAL PLAN

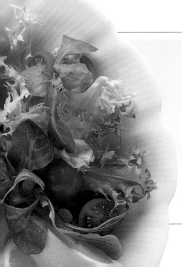

BREAKFAST
Branflakes and raisins with milk; sardines and grilled tomatoes on wholemeal toast; grapefruit juice

MIDMORNING SNACK
Fruit milkshake

LUNCH
Broccoli and sunflower seed soup; wholemeal turkey and watercress sandwich; peach

AFTERNOON SNACK
Watermelon juice; ten cashew nuts and a banana

DINNER
Carrot juice; wholewheat pasta with meat/lentil bolognese and grated cheese; rocket and walnut salad

BEDTIME SNACK
Rest of broccoli soup with wholemeal bread and butter

Exercise Plan

BY NOW YOU WILL BE STARTING TO FOCUS on the birth. Exercise will depend on how you are feeling. As your weight increases, your centre of gravity moves back, and your uterus enlarges, you may find it harder to exercise. You may prefer to concentrate on gentle stretching, walking, swimming and breathing exercises.

GENERAL GUIDELINES

You should at all times be aware of general guidelines relating to exercise during pregnancy (*see pages 18–19*). It is especially important to warm up before doing any form of exercise and to cool down when you have finished (*see page 32*).

EXERCISING FOR LABOUR

Exercises in the third trimester can help you to prepare for labour. You can also practise positions that both strengthen key muscles and joints ready for giving birth and can be used during labour. Include these positions in your exercise programme in the last trimester.
• **Tailor sitting** (*see right*) Sit on the floor with the soles of your feet together and your back straight. Pull the heels as close to your body as you can without strain. Pull one leg into position at a time, and release it before bringing the other leg up, to avoid putting excessive pressure on the symphysis pubic joint.

• **Squatting** This exercise helps to open up the pelvic outlet, encouraging the baby's head to become engaged (*see pages 70–1*), and to improve the flexibility of the pelvic joints, knees and ankles. Do not take up this position for more than a couple of minutes at a time, however, since it may restrict the circulation of blood to the legs. Also, it is advisable to warm up in a particular way before doing squats.
• **Warm up for squatting** Stand with your hands against a wall for support. Do heel raises to contract the calf muscles before they are stretched during squats
• **Sitting squats** Place a stool against the wall and stand with your back to it, feet hip-width apart and slightly turned out. Keeping the feet flat on the floor, slowly lower your body down so that you are sitting on the stool. Use a nearby door handle or piece of furniture to help you to keep your balance as you go down. You can also practise squatting using a chair for support if you prefer (*see opposite*).

TAILOR SITTING
This position promotes flexibility around the hip joints by stretching the muscle of the inner thigh.

SQUATTING

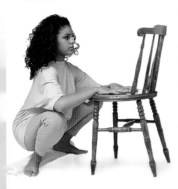

USING A CHAIR
Stand facing a chair with the feet hip-width apart and slightly turned out. Slowly bend the knees, lowering yourself into a full squat, keeping the knees in line with the feet, which remain flat, and holding on to the chair for support. Hold the squatting position for a few seconds, then straighten up. Repeat two or three times.

STRENGTHENING THE PELVIC FLOOR

The pelvis is cleverly designed to ease your baby's exit from the uterus when the time comes. The joints of the pelvis are softened during pregnancy by hormonal action, increasing their elasticity and ability to allow movement as the baby progresses down the birth canal. The pelvic floor itself resembles a sling of muscle, attached to the pelvic bone at the front and passing in two halves to the sacrum and coccyx at the back. The two halves fan out to form the floor of the pelvis and support the organs in the pelvic cavity. The urethra, vagina and rectum pass through the pelvic floor. The pelvic floor muscles are stretched and weakened in pregnancy, and this can cause urine leakage. Exercises to strengthen these muscles, and especially in the weeks leading up to the birth, will help to prevent this and will also assist you during delivery: exercised muscles stretch and recoil more easily. You can start to do pelvic floor exercises right from the first trimester if you like. You will certainly be advised to continue doing them after the birth of your baby to help to prevent stress incontinence. In fact, women are encouraged to make them part of their exercise programme for the rest of their lives in order to avoid stress incontinence and other problems. Pelvic floor exercises can be done standing, sitting or lying down, wherever you are, and the more often you practise them the better. A good tip to remember to do them regularly is to associate them with another activity that you do regularly such as brushing your teeth, sitting at a red traffic light or watching the news.

• **Pelvic floor exercises** Tighten the ring of muscles around the anus and the vagina, drawing them up inside you as if you were trying to stop a flow of urine. Hold for six seconds and release. Repeat ten times, preferably more, twice a day. Breathe normally throughout. Alternatively, tighten the muscles in four or five stages, rather like a lift ascending one floor at a time. Lower the "lift" in the same way.

STRENGTHENING LEGS

LOAD-BEARING LEGS
The legs carry extra weight during pregnancy so they need to be strong. As your weight increases, exercises that you do to strengthen the lower body (see page 33) will have greater effect. They will also improve circulation and reduce the possibility of swelling in the last weeks of pregnancy.

STRETCHING OUT
Stretch out after exercising using calf stretches. Stand leaning against a wall using your arms, with elbows slightly bent. Put one foot in front of the other. Hold for five seconds. Repeat with the other foot in front.

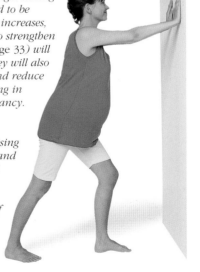

THIRD TRIMESTER

THIRD TRIMESTER

Five-point Action Plan

THE FINAL 12-WEEK PERIOD of your pregnancy is an important preparation time in which to gear yourself up for the birth of your baby. Your body is changing to cope with the growing baby and in preparation for labour and breastfeeding, while the baby is doubling in size as its body systems mature and it lays down stores of fat, iron and calcium.

REST WHENEVER POSSIBLE

While you are resting, the muscles around the uterus relax, increasing blood flow and oxygen supply to your baby. It is difficult to get enough rest if you work late into pregnancy. It is important to put your feet up whenever you can, but especially between 3 pm and 5 pm. Working too hard and for too long during the third trimester may inhibit your baby's growth. Women who go into labour feeling tired are likely to have a more difficult time than those who are rested.

BOOST ENERGY

Your metabolism becomes more efficient over this period in order to provide extra nutrients for the baby and to prepare your body for labour. You will need about 200 extra calories a day, and protein requirements are at an all-time high. It is also important to drink plenty of water: too little will diminish your energy, undermine your mood and reduce the efficiency of digestion and waste removal.

GEAR UP MENTALLY

In order to prepare yourself, not just for the birth of your baby but for life thereafter as a parent, it is important take time to sit quietly, breathe deeply and contemplate. Everyone expects a pregnancy to last 40 weeks, and mental preparation is often put off until just before the due date. If labour begins prematurely, you may feel unprepared, which could affect you negatively after the birth. Find 30 minutes every day for some visualization and positive thought.

FEED THE BRAIN

Your baby's brain has its main growth spurt during this period, quadrupling in weight and using two-thirds of the energy supply. Sixty per cent of the brain's structure is made up of fat and essential fatty acids. The baby takes essential fatty acids from your bloodstream via the placenta, and levels in the baby's blood will be twice as high as yours. It is important that you consume plenty of fish oils to improve the cognitive functions of the baby's brain.

CARE FOR THE PERINEUM

Research suggests that if you massage the perineum with natural plant oils, such as wheatgerm, in the weeks leading up to labour, it will help to increase the elasticity and flexibility of the tissues in this area of the body. This may prevent the need for an episiotomy and reduce the risk of tearing in the second stage of labour. Massage the perineum for between 5 and ten minutes a day from 34 weeks onwards.

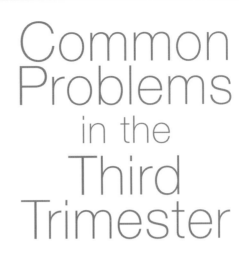

Common Problems in the Third Trimester

MANY OF YOU will still be working but feeling large and uncomfortable. Plenty of rest is important at this stage and, together with complementary therapies, may help to relieve common ailments.

THIRD TRIMESTER

Sleeplessness

SLEEPING DIFFICULTIES are common during pregnancy and lead to fatigue during the day. In early pregnancy, low blood sugar levels as a result of hunger or nausea may cause insomnia. As pregnancy progresses, many women are unable to relax fully in bed due to general discomfort, heartburn, leg cramps or worry about the baby.

SYMPTOMS

Difficulty in falling asleep

✳

Restless, unrefreshing sleep with periods of wakefulness

✳

Fatigue and irritability during the day

MEDITATION

Meditation, particularly Transcendental Meditation, can be used to induce a state of deep relaxation. Studies show that meditation focuses the mind, helping to lower blood pressure, improve brainwave patterns and so encourage sleep. Try to clear your mind of all other matters and focus only on your breathing. Use the following technique:

✳ Find a quiet place where you can meditate without being disturbed. Make yourself comfortable and breathe slowly and regularly for 30 minutes. Try to keep your mind focused on your breathing patterns, and gently refocus your attention if your mind starts to wander. This state of "passive awareness" will make you more conducive to sleep.

See page 143 for further information

POSE FOR THOUGHT
Meditation allows you to concentrate your thoughts in order to calm the mind, relieve tension and induce sleep.

KEY TIPS

Relax before bed and avoid mental stimulation

✳

Try to take regular exercise each day

✳

Avoid drinks containing caffeine in the evening

✳

Eat a substantial lunch and a light supper

✳

Eat calcium and magnesium-rich foods, thought to calm nerves

CAUTION

If sleeplessness persists for longer than two weeks, consult your midwife or doctor because persistent sleep deprivation alters mood.

THIRD TRIMESTER

COMPLEMENTARY TREATMENTS

Before using a complementary treatment, please read any **Cautions** and the relevant page references

ACUPUNCTURE

A practitioner will require details of your sleep patterns. If you cannot sleep between 11 pm and 1 am for example, the peak time for the Gall Bladder meridian, acupuncture points along this meridian will be stimulated to correct any imbalance. Dream-disturbed sleep will also be of interest to a practitioner, since this may indicate a disturbed spirit, or *shen*. Research shows that acupuncture helps to increase production of the neurotransmitter serotonin, which is sometimes deficient in people who have sleeping problems.

See pages 134–5 for further information

SHIATSU

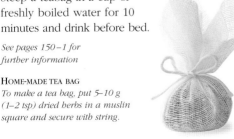

Insomnia is regarded as a disturbance of *shen* (*see above*), and is associated with the Heart meridian. Stimulating the Heart 7 acupoint, located on the inside of the wrists, can help to combat sleeplessness. Apply pressure to the point for 10–15 seconds before you go to bed.

INSOMNIA ACUPOINT
To locate Heart 7, run your finger down from the tip of your little finger to the wrist crease.

See page 138 for further information

WESTERN HERBALISM

There are many herbal teas available that help to relax the nervous system. They include chamomile and lemon balm. Steep a teabag in a cup of freshly boiled water for 10 minutes and drink before bed.

See pages 150–1 for further information

HOME-MADE TEA BAG
To make a tea bag, put 5–10 g (1–2 tsp) dried herbs in a muslin square and secure with string.

AROMATHERAPY

Lavender essential oil, added to a bath or to a carrier oil for massage, can help you to relax. Ask your partner to massage your neck and shoulders gently before you go to bed.

✳ Burn lemon or mandarin oil in a vaporizer; in Traditional Chinese Medicine, mandarin is used to calm the spirit.

Caution: see page 153 for oils to avoid in pregnancy.

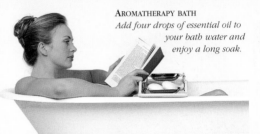

AROMATHERAPY BATH
Add four drops of essential oil to your bath water and enjoy a long soak.

See pages 152–3 for further information

FLOWER REMEDIES

If sleeplessness is due to anxiety, flower remedies may help. Take two drops twice a day in a cup of water, and again before bed. Choice of remedy will depend on symptoms.

✳ Rock rose for any terrifying thoughts.
✳ White chestnut for niggling worries.
✳ Red chestnut to free the mind of negative, fearful thoughts and worries about your baby.

See page 154 for further information

DIET & NUTRITION

Vitamin B deficiency may cause insomnia. If blood sugar levels fall during the night, you may wake because of hunger or nausea.

✳ Calcium-rich foods help to induce sleep by calming the nerves. Eat foods such as almonds, yogurt or sesame seeds as evening snacks.
✳ Foods rich in vitamin B6, such as pulses, green leafy vegetables, nuts, wholegrains and meat have a tranquilizing effect.

See pages 72–3 for further information

THIRD TRIMESTER

Skin Problems

DURING PREGNANCY THE SKIN is affected by hormonal changes. It has to work harder to eliminate toxins and, as the body's shape changes, skin must stretch. Some women experience a marked improvement in skin quality while others develop acne or are plagued by itching. Increased pigmentation occurs in roughly 90 per cent of pregnant women.

SYMPTOMS

Dry, flaky or itchy skin

✻

Acne or blisters

✻

Eczema, dermatitis or psoriasis

✻

Stretch marks

DIET & NUTRITION

The condition of your skin reflects your state of health. A balanced diet helps to protect against skin problems. To maintain skin elasticity, eat plenty of protein and foods containing vitamin C, which also promotes skin health and healing. Drink plenty of water to flush out toxins.

✻ **Dry, flaky skin** may be improved by consuming essential fatty acids, which are found in nuts, seeds and oily fish. Vitamin A, found in carrots, broccoli, sweet potatoes, watercress and melon, and Vitamin B5, in foods such as meat, fish, wholegrains and pulses, also help to combat dry skin. To soothe dry, itchy skin, eat foods containing vitamin B6, such as potatoes, pulses, avocado and cashew nuts.

✻ **Dermatitis**, **acne** and **eczema** can be caused by a deficiency of vitamin B3, which maintains healthy skin. Replenish stocks of this vitamin by eating dairy products, oily fish, poultry, brown rice, yeast extract and nuts.

✻ **Stretch marks** may be prevented by consuming food sources of zinc, such as ginger, cheese and wholegrains.

✻ **Blisters**, cracks around the lips and mouth **eczema** may be due to a deficiency of vitamin B2, which maintains healthy skin and repairs damage. Eat foods such as dark green vegetables, milk, yeast extract, oily fish and sesame seeds.

See pages 72–3 for further information

EATING FRESH FRUIT
A diet that includes lots of vitamin C-rich fresh fruit will help to prevent skin ailments.

CAUTION

If, after 28 weeks, you have very severe itching, consult your doctor in case it is indicative of obstetric cholestasis. This is a serious condition that must be treated with conventional medicine.

KEY TIPS

Drink plenty of water

✻

Avoid sugary foods, animal fats, alcohol and caffeine if you have acne

✻

Avoid stress if you suffer from eczema or psoriasis

THIRD TRIMESTER

COMPLEMENTARY TREATMENTS

Before using a complementary treatment, please read any **Cautions** and the relevant page references

ACUPUNCTURE

According to Traditional Chinese Medicine, itchy skin is caused by excessive "heat" in the Blood. Acupoints are treated to try to clear the heat and alleviate symptoms.

See pages 134–5 for further information

HYDROTHERAPY

To ease **psoriasis**, soak in a warm bath to which soothing oats and lime blossom (which is also available in tea bags) have been added. Place equal quantities of oats and lime blossom in a muslin bag and add to your bath water. Alternatively, add mashed cucumber enclosed in a muslin bag to your bath to soothe and soften the skin. If your skin still feels irritated, soak some cotton wool in fresh cold water and apply to the affected areas after your bath.

See page 144 for further information

HOMEMADE REMEDY
Place oats and lime blossom on a muslin square and tie up to make a little bag.

WESTERN HERBALISM

Herbalism offers plenty of opportunities for treating the irritating skin conditions that are common in pregnancy. Some are soothing applications while others are taken internally.

✱ For **itchy skin**, mix oats with water and gently rub on to the skin as a soothing poultice. Be sure to consult your doctor (see *Caution*, opposite).

✱ For **psoriasis**, drink three cups of dandelion coffee each day, or add a couple of fresh dandelion leaves to a daily salad.

✱ For **acne**, a soothing, healing and anti-inflammatory lotion can be made from lavender, orange blossom and rose petals from a herbal supplier. Infuse 10 g (2 tsp) of each in freshly boiled water and allow the strained liquid to cool before applying it. Use morning and night, storing leftovers in the refrigerator for up to two days.

✱ Also for **acne**, and **eczema**, echinacea is available in tablet form and as a tincture. Follow the manufacturer's

instructions for usage carefully.

✱ For **eczema** arising from nutritional deficiencies, evening primrose oil is beneficial. Your doctor can prescribe capsules, which are the best source. In cases of dry eczema, apply evening primrose oil directly to the skin twice daily.

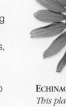
ECHINACEA
This plant has a soothing, cooling effect.

✱ For **dermatitis**, make a cooling spray using warm mineral water and an infusion of chamomile or calendula to alleviate symptoms. This may also relieve **eczema**.

✱ For skin complaints generally, try nettles. Traditionally used for treating skin complaints, they contain many nutrients, including silica, which are beneficial for skin tone. Drink nettle tea by making an infusion from the dried leaves or by using a teabag.

✱ For **stretch marks**, apply calendula cream or cocoa butter, which may help to reduce them.

✱ For **itchy skin**, apply echinacea tincture diluted with water (proportions half and half).

See pages 150–1 for further information

AROMATHERAPY

To treat **acne**, apply diluted tea tree or lavender essential oils, which are antiseptic and may help to reduce inflammation. Carefully dab the oil on to each individual spot with a cotton bud, taking care not to spread oil all over the whole of the area affected by acne. Do not continue this treatment indefinitely: try it for a week or two, stop it for a couple of weeks, then resume. If symptoms persist, maintain this intermittent cycle of treatment. For other skin conditions, try the following.

✱ Massage the skin with a gentle oill such as mandarin in a carrier oil such as wheatgerm. This may help to reduce **stretch marks**.

Caution: some oils may be unsuitable for eczema and dermatitis; see page 153 for oils to avoid in pregnancy.

See pages 152–3 for further information

THIRD TRIMESTER

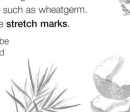

Stress & Anxiety

PREGNANCY is one of the greatest changes a woman undergoes in life, and change is nearly always accompanied by stress. As well as the physical stresses of fatigue, nausea and altered body shape, you may feel anxious about being pregnant, about finances or the baby's health. Prolonged stress can affect mother and baby adversely, so try to find ways to relax.

SYMPTOMS

Insomnia
*
*Rapid, shallow
breathing*
*
Increased metabolic rate
*
Muscle tension

RELAXATION

Relaxation techniques, such as deep breathing, are valuable in the third trimester when tiredness and anxiety about the birth test your ability to cope. While everyday stress does not affect your baby, if you are in a permanent state of anxiety, stress hormones constantly circulate in your body and may cross the placenta. Unremitting stress raises blood pressure. Breathing exercises help to generate alpha brainwaves which are associated with calm and deep relaxation.

✱ To practise deep breathing, lie on the floor or sit comfortably, placing one hand on your chest and one on your stomach (*see page 36*). Inhale and exhale slowly, aiming to take between 12 and 15 breaths a minute. Listening to music may relax you further.

See also page 142–3

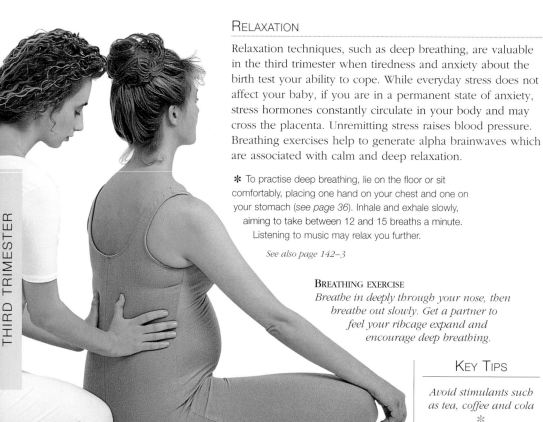

BREATHING EXERCISE
Breathe in deeply through your nose, then breathe out slowly. Get a partner to feel your ribcage expand and encourage deep breathing.

THIRD TRIMESTER

KEY TIPS

Avoid stimulants such as tea, coffee and cola
*
Eat foods that release fuel slowly, keeping blood sugar levels stable
*
Avoid sugary foods, which only provide short-term energy bursts
*
Make time for yourself and talk about anxieties

CAUTION

There are degrees of stress and anxiety. Talk to your midwife or doctor if you are concerned that your stress levels may be adversely affecting you or your baby.

COMPLEMENTARY TREATMENTS

Before using a complementary treatment, please read any **Cautions** and the relevant page references

REIKI

Reiki is believed to work on the body on a spiritual, mental and physical level. Healing energy is thought to flow through the hands of a practitioner to wherever it is needed in your body, which is deeply relaxing.

See page 139 for further information

MEDITATION

The best form of meditation for stress is Transcendental Meditation. The physiological effects include a drop in your metabolic rate.

See page 143 for further information

COLOUR THERAPY

Colour therapists believe that blue can help to relieve stress, so wear blue clothes or drape a blue sheet or cloth over yourself when doing breathing exercises. Alternatively, imagine yourself absorbing a beneficial colour so that it saturates your body or is directed to where it is needed. Good colours to visualize are red, orange and yellow entering at the feet and green entering at the level of the heart.

See page 145 for further information

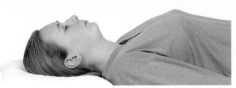

SEEING BLUE
Colour therapists use blue to encourage feelings of calm, relaxation and trust.

WESTERN HERBALISM

Herbs that are believed to combat stress are lemon balm, lime flowers, lavender and chamomile. These can be drunk as teas, and may help to relax the muscles and to lower raised blood pressure levels.

Caution: do not take raspberry leaf in the first trimester since it can stimulate the uterus.

See pages 150–1 for further information

AROMATHERAPY

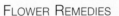

An aromatherapy massage can rid the neck of tension. Beneficial oils include neroli, chamomile, lavender, rose, mandarin and sandalwood. Diffuse calming vapours around a room by putting a few drops of oil in a vaporizer or on a cloth placed on a radiator. Alternatively, add four drops of any of the above oils to your bath water.

Caution: see page 153 for essential oils to avoid in pregnancy.

See pages 152–3 for further information

FLOWER REMEDIES

Flower remedies are especially popular for easing stress and emotional problems.

✱ Red chestnut for fearful, negative thoughts about the baby.

✱ Walnut for coping with adjustments in your life.

✱ Aspen for apprehension.

✱ Rescue Remedy for shock or panic.

See pages 154 for further information

DIET & NUTRITION

Being in a state of stress burns energy and uses up vital nutrients, such as vitamin C, co-enzyme Q10, zinc and magnesium. You may not have much appetite, but it is important to eat foods rich in these nutrients as well as B vitamin, which are needed to release energy. Ensure that you eat plenty of complex carbohydrates, such as wholemeal bread, which release energy slowly, and avoid eating sugary snacks.

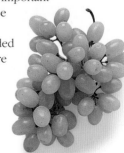

GRAPES
Fruit such as grapes are a good source of vitamin C, a stress-busting nutrient.

See pages 72–3 for further information

THIRD TRIMESTER

Raised Blood Pressure

RAISED BLOOD PRESSURE, or pregnancy-induced hypertension, tends to occur after 20 weeks, and affects 5–10 per cent of women. A blood pressure reading greater than 140 over 90 will cause concern, although there may be no symptoms. First-time mothers, those carrying twins, and very young or older mothers are more likely to have raised blood pressure.

SYMPTOMS OF PRE-ECLAMPSIA

Headaches, nausea and vomiting, oedema
*
Visual disturbances
*
Raised blood pressure, protein in the urine

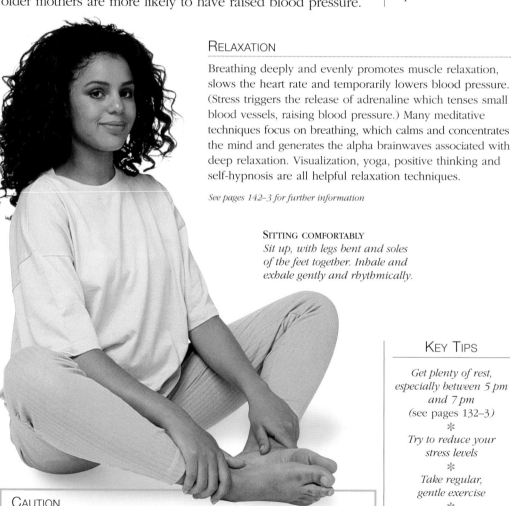

RELAXATION

Breathing deeply and evenly promotes muscle relaxation, slows the heart rate and temporarily lowers blood pressure. (Stress triggers the release of adrenaline which tenses small blood vessels, raising blood pressure.) Many meditative techniques focus on breathing, which calms and concentrates the mind and generates the alpha brainwaves associated with deep relaxation. Visualization, yoga, positive thinking and self-hypnosis are all helpful relaxation techniques.

See pages 142–3 for further information

SITTING COMFORTABLY
Sit up, with legs bent and soles of the feet together. Inhale and exhale gently and rhythmically.

KEY TIPS

*Get plenty of rest, especially between 5 pm and 7 pm
(see pages 132–3)*
*
Try to reduce your stress levels
*
Take regular, gentle exercise
*
Eat a healthy, balanced diet
*
Make sure that you get plenty of sleep

CAUTION

Raised blood pressure can be dangerous for you and the baby if it is left untreated. Consult your doctor if you experience any symptoms of pre-eclampsia (*see above*).

THIRD TRIMESTER

COMPLEMENTARY TREATMENTS

Before using a complementary treatment, please read any **Cautions** and the relevant page references

ACUPUNCTURE

Acupuncture can be of benefit in the treatment of raised blood pressure but in conjunction with conventional medicine. A practitioner will insert needles into the hypertensive point in the ear. A small "patch" can be inserted into this point to facilitate self-help treatment.

See pages 134–5 for further information

SHIATSU

Shiatsu massage on the Pericardium 6 acupoint can help to reduce the stress and anxiety that may be contributing to raised blood pressure.

See page 138 for further information

REFLEXOLOGY

Massaging certain reflex points on the feet may help to lower blood pressure. Consult a qualified practitioner for treatment.

See page 140–1 for further information

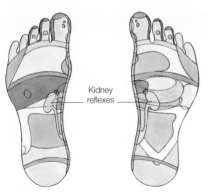

Kidney reflexes

LOWERING BLOOD PRESSURE
Gentle massage of the kidney reflex zones will ease tension and therefore lower blood pressure.

COLOUR THERAPY

Blue is associated with relaxation, and is used therapeutically for the treatment of raised blood pressure. Try lying down beneath a blue sheet or blanket for 20 minutes a day.

See page 145 for further information

HOMEOPATHY

Homeopathic remedies may help to lower blood pressure. A practitioner will prescribe constitutionally, based on your medical history and specific symptoms. You may be given one of the following remedies.

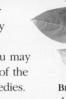

BELLADONNA
A remedy based on this plant is given for a sudden rise in blood pressure.

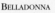

✳ For protein in the urine, swollen hands and feet, irritability and fatigue, *Apis 6c.*

✳ For swelling that is worse for physical exertion, with great thirst, *Natrum mur. 6c.*

✳ For sudden onset, protein in the urine, and symptoms that are worse after 3 pm, *Belladonna 6c.*

See pages 148–9 for dosage and further information

AROMATHERAPY

Massage using any essential oil that an individual finds pleasant may reduce tension and therefore lower blood pressure temporarily. Alternatively, add a few drops of oil to a warm (not hot) bath.

Caution: see page 153 for oils to avoid in pregnancy.

See pages 152–3 for further information

DIET & NUTRITION

Good intakes of vitamins C and E have been found to help women with raised blood pressure. A diet that is low in animal fats but high in fish oils, which help to keep the blood thin, is also recommended. Eat plenty of raw fruit and vegetables, which are rich in vitamin C and potassium, and take 15 ml (1 tbsp) daily of ground linseed, sesame or sunflower seeds for extra calcium and magnesium. Eat garlic regularly to help to lower blood pressure and also to improve blood flow in the placenta.

See pages 72–3 for further information

THIRD TRIMESTER

Oedema, Carpal Tunnel Syndrome & Leg Cramps

OEDEMA, OR MILD SWELLING, of the ankles or hands often occurs in pregnancy, particularly in the third trimester. Carpal tunnel syndrome is caused by swelling of the hands restricting nerves in the wrist. Leg cramps or "restless legs" are often experienced by pregnant women, and usually indicate mineral deficiency.

THIRD TRIMESTER

SYMPTOMS

Swollen ankles or hands (oedema)

✳

Numb, tingling or painful fingers, often worse at night (carpal tunnel syndrome)

✳

Cramp or unpleasant prickling feeling in legs

MASSAGE

Gentle leg massage may help to reduce **oedema**, improve circulation and reduce the risk of **leg cramps**. Use 10 ml (1 tsp) natural plant oil, such as wheatgerm, grapeseed or soya, and slow, repetitive movements to unblock congestion in the lymphatic system and improve blood circulation.

See also pages 152–3

MASSAGE TECHNIQUE
For lymphatic drainage, use skin-deep strokes towards the body. Stroke one hand after the other or place one hand on each side of the leg and stroke both together. Apply greater pressure in order to affect the flow of blood through the veins.

KEY TIPS

Rest with legs elevated for 20 minutes, three or four times a day to reduce swollen ankles

✳

Use pillows to elevate hands and arms when you rest to relieve carpal tunnel syndrome

✳

Stand on the ground and curl your toes to relieve cramp

CAUTIONS

If you have carpal tunnel syndrome, take extra care when handling hot liquids, especially first thing in the morning when symptoms may be worse. If you have severe swelling and a headache, contact your doctor or midwife at once, since this could be a sign of pre-eclampsia.

COMPLEMENTARY TREATMENTS

Before using a complementary treatment, please read any **Cautions** and the relevant page references

ACUPUNCTURE

Acupuncturists believe that **carpal tunnel** swelling is the result of imbalance in the Spleen and Kidney meridians. A practitioner will insert acupuncture needles into the carpal tunnel, angled towards the wrist, and also into the Stomach 36 point below the knee. This usually relieves pain for about 24 hours.

See pages 134–5 for further information

SHIATSU

Stimulating the Pericardium 6 acupoint may relieve pain from swelling. Press firmly three fingers down from the wrist crease between the two tendons for 10–15 seconds at a time.

See page 138 for further information

OSTEOPATHY

To ease swollen hands and **carpal tunnel syndrome**, an osteopath may manipulate the wrist to improve lymphatic drainage. A physiotherapist can provide splints to support the wrists.

CARPAL TUNNEL TREATMENT
An osteopath will encourage the dispersal of excess fluid in the local soft tissue.

✱ Self-help measures for carpal tunnel syndrome include gentle wrist exercises (circling and flexing) in ice-cold water. Alternatively, crouch down and gently press the hands flat on the floor, which stretches the carpal tunnel.

See page 146 for further information

HOMEOPATHY

One of the following homeopathic remedies may be recommended by a practitioner:

✱ For **carpal tunnel syndrome** with a tingling sensation and numbness in the fingers that is better for warmth, *Arsen. alb. 6c*.

✱ For **cramp** that occurs when stretching the legs in bed and that is worse at night, *Calc. carb. 6c*.

See pages 148–9 for dosage and further information

WESTERN HERBALISM

Apply cabbage-leaf poultices to the affected areas to reduce oedema. Herbal teas such as nettle and dandelion have a diuretic effect and stimulate the kidneys to process more fluid. Dandelion

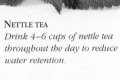

NETTLE TEA
Drink 4–6 cups of nettle tea throughout the day to reduce water retention.

is also a rich source of vitamins A, C and E and the minerals calcium and potassium.

See pages 150–1 for further information

DIET & NUTRITION

To relieve **oedema**, eat onion and garlic, which are good circulatory tonics. Choose foods that are natural diuretics, such as celery, asparagus, artichokes, grapes, blackcurrants and parsley. Vitamin C is a mild diuretic so increase intake of citrus fruits, red berries, peppers and green leafy vegetables. B vitamins are good for the nerves and **carpal tunnel syndrome**. Vitamin B-rich foods include sesame seeds, chickpeas, bananas, yeast extract and hazelnuts. **Leg cramps** can be due to calcium and magnesium deficiencies, so eat milk products and green leafy vegetables (for calcium) and wholegrains, wheatgerm, nuts, seeds, soya, dried apricots and raw green leafy vegetables (for magnesium). Also bear in mind the following:

✱ Avoid refined forms of table salt and use natural sea salt or rock salt from health food shops.

✱ Drink plenty of water.

✱ For cramp, take a bone mineral complex or a supplement of magnesium before bed.

See pages 72–3 for further information

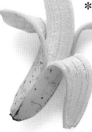

BANANA
The vitamin B⁶ in bananas has a diuretic effect, relieving carpal tunnel syndrome.

THIRD TRIMESTER

Breech Baby

IF YOUR BABY IS IN THE BREECH POSITION, it means that its bottom is lying in the pelvis instead of its head. This occurs in 3–4 per cent of full-term pregnancies: in most cases a breech baby will turn itself before birth, sometimes as late as week 40. If your first baby is in the breech position, you may need to have a Caesarean section delivery.

SYMPTOMS

Feeling the baby's head beneath your ribs

✳

Experiencing the baby kicking in the region of the bladder

ACUPUNCTURE

Moxibustion has been used for centuries in China to turn breech babies. It involves the use of the herb moxa, which is formed into long sticks. The moxa is lit next to significant acupoints, creating a sensation of gentle warmth. The theory behind this practice is that the heat travels up the Bladder meridian, which is linked to the uterus. Moxibustion is most successful if used between 32 and 36 weeks. Increasing numbers of midwives are becoming interested in this technique.

✳ The smouldering end of a moxa stick is held near the acupuncture point on the nail of each little toe for 15 minutes once or twice a day. Your acupuncturist will show you how to do this and will give you some moxa to take home for a partner or friend to apply.

✳ The baby may move while moxibustion takes place, presumably stimulated by the heat. If you feel the baby turn, stop treatment at once and get your midwife to check its position.

Caution: only use this technique if you are healthy, you do not have raised blood pressure and you have not experienced any bleeding.
See also pages 134–5

MOXA STICKS
The heat from moxa sticks may help to turn a breech baby.

KEY TIPS

Only use qualified practitioners and preferably those who have experience of treating pregnant women

CAUTION

Check with your midwife before using natural remedies in case there is a significant reason for your baby being breech. Only try natural remedies if you are healthy, are not carrying twins and have never had a Caesarean section.

THIRD TRIMESTER

COMPLEMENTARY TREATMENTS

Before using a complementary treatment, please read any **Cautions** and the relevant page references

YOGA

Use inverted yoga positions – that is, those in which your head is level with or lower than the rest of your body, such as the Cat pose – in an attempt to discourage the baby's head from settling in the pelvis and so move into a head-down position. (The head is the heaviest part of the baby.) Alternatively, place a wooden board at an angle of 45º with one end on the floor and the other resting on a chair. The board should be long and wide enough to support you securely. Lie on it with your head at the floor end. Spend 15–20 minutes each day in this position or lying on the floor with two pillows beneath your back so that the hips are higher than the shoulders and your legs are up against a wall at a 45º-degree angle. Relax and concentrate on your baby moving into the correct position (*see also* Visualization, *right*). In addition to

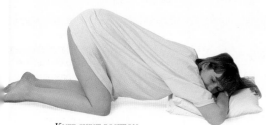

KNEE-CHEST POSITION
Use a pillow to rest your head so that you can maintain this position comfortably.

recognized yoga positions, try the following measures to encourage your baby to move.

✻ Kneel on the floor with your bottom in the air and your head on the floor, resting on your arms (*see above*). Stay in this knee-chest position for about 10–15 minutes each day.

✻ Sleep with several pillows under your bottom and lower back to allow gravity to help to turn the baby for an extended period while you are sleeping.

✻ Any activity that involves getting down on your hands and knees may encourage the baby to dislodge from its bottom-down position.

See page 142 for further information

VISUALIZATION

Spend some time each day imagining that your baby's head is presented (that is, in the correct position to emerge first). Try to relax fully, either on a bed or in a comfortable chair, and attempt to transfer thoughts to your baby about why you want it to move into a head-down position. If you like, you can gently massage your stomach at the same time with a little natural plant oil, such as wheatgerm, since this aids relaxation.

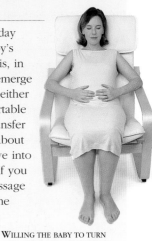

WILLING THE BABY TO TURN
Relax somewhere comfortable every day and imagine your baby changing its position.

See page 143 for further information

EXERCISE

Walking for about 20 minutes each day may encourage your baby to move so that the head presents downwards. In addition to your usual exercise routine:

✻ Regularly take up upright, forward-leaning positions from week 34 onwards. This will tilt the pelvis forwards, giving the baby slightly more room to manoeuvre.

See pages 74–5 for further information

HOMEOPATHY

Pulsatilla 30c has traditionally been prescribed to encourage breech babies or babies in the transverse position to turn. It is, however, advisable to consult a fully qualified homeopathic practitioner before taking any remedies for a breech baby. You may need to be treated constitutionally.

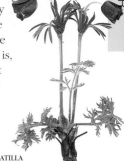

PULSATILLA
The remedy based on this plant is believed to encourage a baby to turn.

See pages 148–9 for further information

THIRD TRIMESTER

Respiratory Problems

FROM EARLY PREGNANCY, the lungs and diaphragm become compressed in order to accommodate the expanding uterus. Breathing becomes shallower, and any respiratory weakness, such as a tendency to hayfever, may worsen. You may also find yourself more prone to respiratory infections, which can be exacerbated by a poor diet that is full of additives.

SYMPTOMS

Streaming eyes, running or blocked nose

✻

Sore throat, hoarseness, loss of voice, cough

✻

Breathing difficulties, fever, pain

INHALATING VAPOURS
Essential oils, inhaled in steam, can ease respiratory problems. A towel over the head helps to trap the steam.

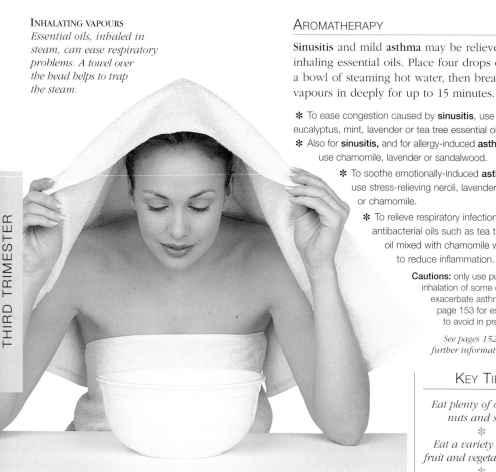

AROMATHERAPY

Sinusitis and mild **asthma** may be relieved by inhaling essential oils. Place four drops of oil in a bowl of steaming hot water, then breathe the vapours in deeply for up to 15 minutes.

✻ To ease congestion caused by **sinusitis**, use eucalyptus, mint, lavender or tea tree essential oils.

✻ Also for **sinusitis,** and for allergy-induced **asthma**, use chamomile, lavender or sandalwood.

✻ To soothe emotionally-induced **asthma**, use stress-relieving neroli, lavender, rose, or chamomile.

✻ To relieve respiratory infections, use antibacterial oils such as tea tree. This oil mixed with chamomile will help to reduce inflammation.

Cautions: only use pure oils; inhalation of some oils may exacerbate asthma; see page 153 for essential oils to avoid in pregnancy.

See pages 152–3 for further information

KEY TIPS

Eat plenty of oily fish, nuts and seeds

✻

Eat a variety of fresh fruit and vegetables daily

✻

Cut down on animal fats and dairy products

✻

Avoid foods laden with additives, preservatives or artificial colourants

THIRD TRIMESTER

CAUTIONS

Consult your doctor before taking natural remedies for asthma. Do not stop taking prescribed medication. For bronchitis, see your doctor immediately.

COMPLEMENTARY TREATMENTS

Before using a complementary treatment, please read any **Cautions** and the relevant page references

ACUPUNCTURE

In Traditional Chinese Medicine, **hayfever** is regarded as an invasion of "heat" and "wind", and can be treated at acupoints on the back. Treating points on the Lung and Kidney meridians may help those with **asthma**.

See pages 134–5 for further information

YOGA

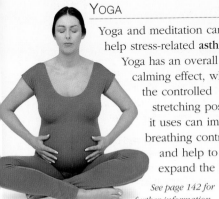

Yoga and meditation can help stress-related **asthma**. Yoga has an overall calming effect, while the controlled stretching postures it uses can improve breathing control and help to expand the lungs.

See page 142 for further information

DEEP BREATHING
Sitting comfortably and concentrating on deep breathing induces calm and improves technique.

ALEXANDER TECHNIQUE

The improved posture taught by an Alexander teacher may reduce the shoulder hunching that is common to many people with **asthma**.

See page 147 for further information

HOMEOPATHY

A number of self-help remedies can be used to treat **hayfever**, depending on the precise nature of your symptoms:

✱ For burning eyes, frequent sneezing, runny nose, puffy eyelids and exhaustion, *Arsen. alb. 6c.*

✱ For burning nasal **catarrh**, sneezing and eye inflammation, *Allium cepa 6c.*

✱ For itchy ears, stuffy nose, inflamed eyes and watery catarrh, *Euphrasia 6c.*

✱ For chronic **rhinitis**, *Nux vomica. 6c.*

See pages 148–9 for dosage and further information

WESTERN HERBALISM

A number of herbs help to relieve respiratory problems. Steep 5–10 g (1–2 tsp) dried herb in 250 ml (9 fl oz) freshly boiled water for about 10 minutes, then drink. Take three times a day. Some herbs can be used in cooking.

✱ To ease **asthma**, try ginger, German chamomile, elderflower, nettle or thyme. Capsules of evening primrose oil may help some types of asthma, particularly if it is allergy-related.

✱ To soothe **bronchitis**, use thyme or ginger. Garlic and onions, eaten raw if possible, have good antibacterial properties.

✱ To clear **catarrhal** congestion, sip elderflower tea or 1 tbsp (15 ml) cider vinegar in hot water. Alternatively, make an infusion of thyme.

✱ To ease mild **hayfever**, drink tea made from chamomile, lavender, nettle, or take dandelion root tincture.

See pages 150–1 for further information

DIET & NUTRITION

Oily fish are rich in omega-3 fatty acids, which may alleviate inflammation and allergic reactions. Vitamin E and selenium are good anti-inflammatories, and are found in cold-pressed oils, green leafy vegetables, nuts and sunflower seeds. Vitamin C (found in foods such as broccoli, tomatoes, peppers and citrus fruit) is an antihistamine. Follow these other dietary guidelines:

✱ To prevent respiratory ailments from being exacerbated by dairy products, limit your intake but supplement your diet with calcium-rich alternatives such as sesame seeds, broccoli, tofu, sardines or watercress.

✱ To ease **asthma**, eliminate foods that you are allergic to while maintaining a balanced diet. In general, lower your fat intake and increase your fish and fruit consumption.

✱ To relieve severe **hayfever**, take vitamin C and pantothenic acid supplements.

See pages 72–3 for further information

THIRD TRIMESTER

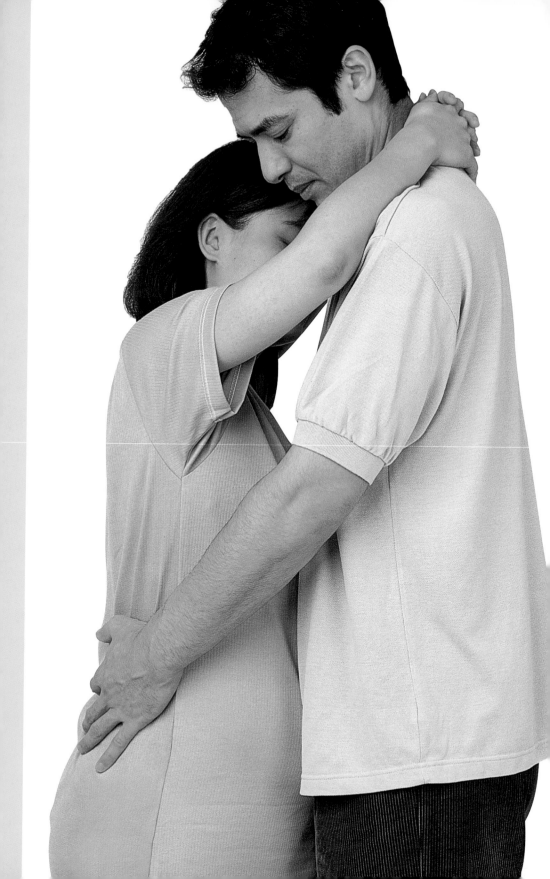

WHEN YOU THINK ABOUT LABOUR during pregnancy, it is probably with a mixture of apprehension and fear. Acquainting yourself with the stages and common behaviour patterns of labour, however, is useful preparation for the event. This chapter provides a sort of "ready, steady, go" countdown to labour, describing signs

Preparation for labour & baby

to expect, nutrition in the run-up to the birth, natural methods of pain relief and induction and practical tips to help you prepare physically and mentally. It guides you through the stages of labour, explaining some of the feelings you may experience and what will be happening to your body and the baby so that you will know exactly what to expect when it happens and how to help yourself.

The Vital Link

ATTACHED TO THE WALL of the uterus, the placenta connects you to your baby via the umbilical cord and supplies all the baby's needs while it is in the womb. Beginning as a small cluster of cells, the placenta becomes deeply embedded in the uterine wall as it grows and develops ever more complex functions.

KEY TIPS

Eat a balanced diet

✳

Give up work by 32–34 weeks

✳

Get as much rest, relaxation and sleep as you can

✳

Reduce your stress levels

A UNIQUE ORGAN

At the birth of your baby, the placenta consists of a flat, round or oval disk, 18–20 cm (7–8 in) in diameter, and 2.5 cm (1 in) thick. It weighs about 600 g (20 oz) – roughly one-sixth of the weight of the baby. The maternal surface of the placenta has 15–20 lobes, which are called cotyledons. The foetal side has the umbilical cord growing out of the centre of it, with blood vessels radiating from it. The umbilical cord is about 50 cm (20 in) in length, 2 cm (¾ in) in thickness and is composed of a jelly-like substance.

PLACENTAL FUNCTIONS

As it develops, the placenta takes over the key functions that sustain the pregnancy.
• It produces vital hormones. One of these, human chorionic gonadotrophin (HCG), starts circulating in your blood from the moment that you conceive.
• The placenta prevents you from rejecting the baby by separating your bloodstream from that of the baby by means of a membrane. Your blood does not flow directly into the baby but diffuses through this membrane. The baby's blood diffuses back the other way.
• The placenta provides oxygen and removes waste. The umbilical cord has one blood vessel that carries oxygen and nutrients to the baby and two that carry carbon dioxide and waste products away. Blood flows through the placenta at the rate of 36 litres (8 gal) a day at 16 weeks. This increases to 455 litres (100 gal) a day at full term.
• It provides all the baby's nutritional needs: proteins for growth; glucose for energy; essential fatty acids for brain development; and water. Taking what the baby needs from your blood, the placenta uses some substances straight

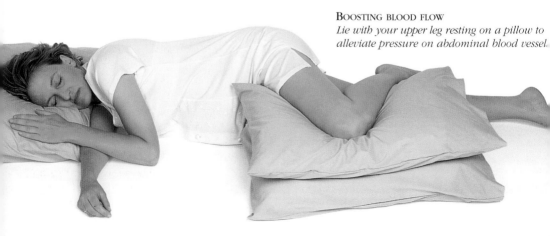

BOOSTING BLOOD FLOW
Lie with your upper leg resting on a pillow to alleviate pressure on abdominal blood vessel.

way, stores some and modifies others so that they can be used by the baby.
● The placenta acts as a barrier, preventing the passage of bacteria, viruses and micro-organisms, while allowing the transfer of antibodies that give the baby immunity. It does not, however, prevent the passage of alcohol, which enters the baby's bloodstream in the same concentration as it is in yours.

MATERNAL NUTRITION

A well-nourished woman usually develops a healthy placenta. Despite a good supply of nutrients, a baby can become undernourished if the transportation of nutrients across the placenta is inadequate. Iron is needed by the mother to expand her blood volume and by the baby to establish good levels of haemoglobin. If iron levels fall, the efficiency of red blood cells in carrying oxygen is reduced and tissues become deficient in energy.

Zinc is stored in the placenta. High zinc levels are associated with a greater birth weight.
● Vitamin E, gingko biloba and co-enzyme Q10 are all thought to improve blood supply.

BOOSTING THE PLACENTA

Improve the efficiency of the placenta by:
● **Eating a balanced diet** Good nutrition is vital for a healthy placenta.
● **Resting as much as possible** Relax the muscles, particularly the abdominals, thereby increasing blood flow to the placenta. Choose

---

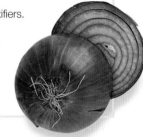

DETOXIFYING THE BODY

Research suggests that the placenta does not block the passage of certain toxins to the baby. To help to protect yourself and the baby, eat the following foods/nutrients:

● Garlic, onion, bananas, apples and pears to reduce absorption of toxins generally.
● Beans, peas and lentils, which act as detoxifiers.
● B vitamins for general protection.
● Vitamin C and zinc to reduce levels of lead in the blood; vitamin E to reduce the risk of lead poisoning; and calcium to prevent the absorption of lead.

---

a comfortable position and practise deep breathing and visualization (*see pages 143*) for at least 30 minutes a day during the third trimester. Imagine that stress and tension are leaving your body as you exhale, and that oxygen is filling your lungs and blood and reaching the baby via the placenta as you inhale.
● **Sleeping** Most cell repair and cell growth takes place when you are asleep.
● **Giving up work** You should have stopped work by about weeks 32–34. To maintain

VITAMIN E
This is needed for good blood circulation.

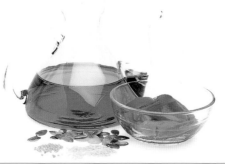

an adequate blood supply to the baby via the placenta, you must have plenty of rest in the last two months of pregnancy. Stress causes blood vessels to constrict, restricting flow. Working too hard may cause premature birth and reduce the baby's weight at birth.

CAUSES OF PROBLEMS

Problems with the placenta can be caused by raised blood pressure, severe anaemia, stress, tobacco, caffeine, alcohol, and overwork and lack of rest. Your midwife will assess at antenatal visits whether or not your abdomen is small for your dates. Tests can detect placental malfunction. A Doppler ultrasound measures blood flow in the umbilical artery and checks for intra-uterine growth retardation (whereby the baby's growth slows because of oxygen starvation). Placenta previa means that the placenta overlaps the cervix (diagnosed by ultrasound scan). The placenta usually moves up as the pregnancy progresses.

Countdown to Labour

IN THE LAST FEW WEEKS before your baby is born it will help you mentally to know that you are taking positive steps towards the event. It is not easy to think beyond labour, especially if this is your first baby and you are, understandably, feeling apprehensive.

KEY TIPS

Rest as much as possible
✳
Eat what your body tells you to and drink plenty of fresh water

THE LAST FEW WEEKS OF PREGNANCY

WEEK 34

✳ You will have started antenatal classes.
✳ Make sure you have an adequate night's sleep and two hours' rest in the afternoon.
✳ Exercise three times a week to suit you (*see pages 18–19 and 74–5*).
✳ Visualize your baby and communicate positive thoughts (*see right and page 143*).
✳ Eat iron-rich foods (*see pages 13*).
✳ Daily massage of the perineum before the birth may help to prevent tears. Soak in a bath to soften the area. Place natural plant oil on your thumb or index finger and place in the vagina at least 5 cm (2 in), pressing towards the rectum. Gently stretch the area in a U-shaped motion until you feel a tingling sensation. Release and massage. Repeat for five to ten minutes.
✳ Start taking raspberry leaf, either as tea or tablets, to help to tone the uterus.

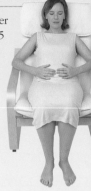

WEEK 35

✳ Go over the Shiatsu points for labour with your partner.
✳ Do some pelvic floor exercises (*see page 75*) every day. Toning the muscles of the pelvic floor will help them to stretch and recoil more easily during and after the birth, and will also help to prevent the leakage of urine after the birth.
✳ Exercise gently for a little while every day. Swimming, walking and yoga are good at this stage.
✳ Practise gentle stretching that will help to prepare your pelvis for labour, such as tailor sitting (*see left and page 74*).

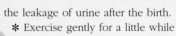

WEEK 36

✳ You may start to feel fed up with being pregnant, especially if you are tired, uncomfortable and sleeping badly. Have a relaxing aromatherapy massage.
✳ Mugwort flower remedy may encourage the baby to engage (*see page 154*).
✳ Try olive flower remedy if you are exhausted, hornbeam if you are doubting your ability to cope or mimulus if you are beginning to feel afraid.
✳ For an uplifting effect, use frankincense or lemon oil in a vaporizer (*see pages 152–3*).

WEEK 37

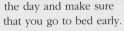

❋ Labour could happen at any time, and you may be feeling anxious. Keep practising your relaxation techniques.

❋ Rest is more important than ever. Put your feet up for a couple of hours during the day and make sure that you go to bed early.

❋ Practise massage techniques with a partner.

❋ Take vitamin C and zinc, both necessary for hormone production prior to delivery.

WEEK 38

❋ Start to eat a diet that is rich in carbohydrates (*see pages 98–9*).

❋ In the ten days before your due date, take the homeopathic remedy *Caulophylum 30c* each night before you go to bed for a week and *Caulophylum 200c* for the last three days. This will help to relieve the pain of contractions. It is best to consult a homeopath (*see pages 148–9*).

❋ Increase your intake of raspberry leaf tea to four cups a day.

❋ Eat plenty of magnesium- and calcium-rich foods to fortify the muscles ready for contractions during labour.

WEEK 39

❋ Co-enzyme Q10 improves the ability of muscles cells to use oxygen and metabolize energy (*see page 99*). Take as a supplement or eat rich food sources.

❋ Eat plenty of foods rich in vitamin K, which is vital for blood clotting (*see page 98*) for you and the baby.

❋ Start taking the homeopathic remedy *Arnica 6c* to help to prevent bruising after the birth (*see pages 148–9*).

WEEK 40

❋ Delivery should be any day now. Start to use acupressure (*see page 136*) and/or a TENS machine (*see page 109*) daily on acupoints LI 4 on the hand (to relieve anxiety and abdominal discomfort) and Sp 6 on the lower leg (to reduce haemorrhaging and strengthen the uterus) ready for labour.

❋ Drink fennel tea to increase milk flow ready for breastfeeding.

❋ Continue to practise positions for labour.

❋ Rest when you can and use the time to practise relaxation techniques (*see below*).

RELAXATION

Prop yourself up and support your knees with pillows when you lie on your back. Do not lie flat on your back at this stage of pregnancy, which might restrict oxygen supply to the baby.

Nutrition during Labour

YOU SHOULD PREPARE YOURSELF FOR LABOUR as if you were in training for a marathon – at least in terms of energy requirements. Building up energy ready for labour will help to prevent tiredness, dehydration, weakness and demoralization, all of which increase the likelihood of medical intervention in the birth.

KEY TIPS

Eat small meals, not large ones, if your stomach feels restricted

✳

Build up energy supplies by eating plenty of carbohydrates

✳

Have snack foods at your disposal during labour

KEY NUTRIENTS

During the last few weeks of pregnancy you should build on the preceding months of healthy eating so that you are prepared for the rigours of labour. Vitamin K is needed in particular to control blood clotting, prevent haemorrhaging and help to heal the placental site. It is derived naturally from bacteria in the mother's gut and supplemented from rich food sources such as broccoli, beans, spinach, avocado, watercress, lettuce, cabbage and cauliflower. A baby's gut is sterile, however, so an infant depends on its mother for vitamin K, before birth via the placenta and after

through breast milk. (Babies may be given vitamin K orally at birth.) Zinc is another very important mineral in the run-up to labour. It is needed to encourage hormone production and healing after the birth.

PRODUCING ENERGY

Simple carbohydrates, which are basic sugars, are quickly absorbed from the digestive system into the bloodstream. Excess glucose in the blood is stored as glycogen in the liver and muscles. When cells need energy, they use the glucose in the blood. If the blood sugar level is low, energy is obtained from glycogen – the longterm

energy reserve. To maintain energy levels, you need to keep your blood sugar level constant by eating complex carbohydrates, which break down gradually and release their sugar content slowly. To ensure that glycogen reserves are filled to capacity, stock up on complex carbohydrates during the two weeks before the birth. This means eating lots of vegetables, wholegrains and pulses. In addition to complex carbohydrates, certain enzymes are needed for energy production. These in turn are dependant on vitamins and minerals. If these are deficient, you will not maximize your

ESSENTIAL DIETARY NUTRIENTS

B vitamins, including folate
Vitamin C
Iron
Calcium
Magnesium
Zinc
Chromium

VEGETABLE SOUP
You may not feel like a full meal as you approach labour, but a "big soup" – with a variety of vegetables, beans and ham in this case – is very nutritious.

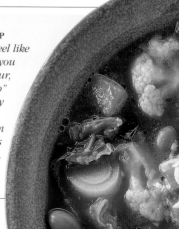

energy potential. To convert glucose into energy, you need:
• B vitamins (B^1, B^2, B^3, B^4, B^6, B^{12}). Sources: meat, poultry, milk, eggs, vegetables, watercress, pulses, nuts, wholegrains. B vitamins include folate. Sources: broccoli, spinach, wheatgerm, seeds, nuts.
• Vitamin C. Sources: citrus fruit, blackcurrants, peppers, broccoli, tomatoes.
• Iron. Sources: pumpkin seeds, prunes, nuts, parsley, apricots.
• Choline, an organic substance needed for the transmission of signals between muscles and nerves during energy production. Sources: eggs, fish, soya beans, wholegrains, nuts, pulses.
• Calcium and magnesium, for maximizing the efficiency of contractions during labour. Sources: cheese, milk, parsley, seeds, beans, nuts, raisins.
• Chromium, for maintaining balanced blood sugar levels. Sources: potatoes, wholemeal bread, peppers, eggs, chicken.
• Co-enzyme Q10, for energy metabolism and the efficient use of oxygen by muscle cells. Sources: meat, fish, eggs, soya beans, spinach, broccoli, alfalfa.

Fuel During Labour

Until recently it was common practice not to eat or drink during labour in case medical intervention requiring the use of anaesthetic was necessary. Anaesthetic carries with it the risk of Mendelson's syndrome, whereby food may be regurgitated and acidic gastric juices inhaled, causing the potentially fatal respiratory distress syndrome. Feeling hungry and thirsty during labour, however, can also have detrimental effects. A lack of energy can slow down the progress of labour, reducing the efficiency of uterine contractions and making medical intervention more likely. If carbohydrates are not available and blood glucose and glycogen supplies are depleted, ketones begin to be produced as the body metabolizes fat stores. Ketones are organic substances that make blood more acidic and less able to transport oxygen efficiently. If you do not drink plenty of fluids during labour then you may become dehydrated, which will also

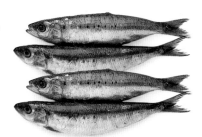

SARDINES
These fish are a good source of protein, calcium and other valuable nutrients.

adversely affect your energy levels. At worst, you may need an intravenous drip, which will greatly restrict your movements during labour. Ideally, you need an energy drink that is specifically designed for the extraordinary demands made upon your body during the often long hours of labour (isotonic sports drinks are not recommended). A combination of maltodextrin and fructose will ensure a sustained energy release, with glucose instantly available and a supply of micronutrients to help your body to metabolize energy efficiently. There are some specially formulated drinks available for this purpose.

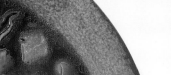

Foods to Fuel Labour

SMALL MEALS & SNACKS
• Small jacket potato
• Sandwiches
• Sardines on toast
• Cold pasta salad
• Rice salad
• Tabbouleh
• Bowl of cereal
• Dried fruit such as apricots
• Banana
• Apple and orange segments

• Grapes
• Celery sticks
• Cheese and biscuits
• Carrot sticks
• Bread sticks
• Crackers
• Cereal bars
• Nuts and raisins

Preparing the Mind

YOUR FRAME OF MIND can greatly enhance the progress of your labour and help to alleviate pain. The more relaxed you are the better. Mental preparation, for which you need adequate time, also helps you to adjust quicker to life after the birth. This is especially important if you are expecting your first baby.

PREPARATION TIME

Given the choice, most women would probably opt for time off after their baby is born rather than in the run-up to the birth. Working until just before the birth, however, means that you might go into labour mentally unprepared and physically exhausted, and it might take far longer to adjust and recover after the birth. Although pregnancy technically lasts for 40 weeks, labour may begin any time after 37 weeks, and giving up work at 32–34 weeks is highly recommended.

VOICING CONCERNS

If this is your first baby, or if you have had a difficult time with a previous birth, you may view labour with a great deal of apprehension. You may have specific fears about tearing, coping with pain or a general fear of the unknown or of something being wrong with the baby. It is important to admit to these fears and try to deal with them in advance, so that during labour you only have to think about what is actually happening to you.

BUILDING CONFIDENCE

Fear can slow your labour right down. Remember that a woman's body is designed for childbirth. The pelvis is the right shape to allow a baby to pass through, and the ligaments are built to stretch. So start your labour from a position of confidence and positive thoughts. Think of your birth plan as an action plan! Assemble your complementary therapies

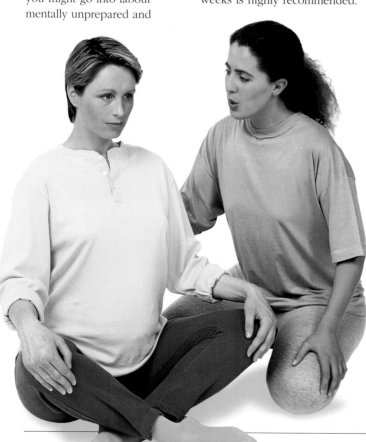

ANTENATAL CLASSES
These give you and your birth partner the opportunity to practise working as a team.

nd plan with your partner which should be used when. Mark up acupressure points, practise using a TENS machine (see page 109) and make sure you are comfortable in the positions that you would like to adopt during labour and birth. Take note of the patterns of behaviour that you may develop during labour so that neither of you will be alarmed if they happen. Do not persuade a male partner to be with you during labour against his will. Support is obviously of great value but not if your partner is reluctant and feels pressurized. This will lead to feelings of inadequacy and possible tension between you later. Consider asking a close female friend instead, or anyone who you feel you can trust to give you the support you need.

MEDITATION & VISUALIZATION

Try to find a little time every day to sit quietly alone and clear your mind. Make yourself comfortable, close your eyes and focus on your breathing. Inhale and exhale slowly and naturally: just observe how you breathe rather than trying to change it. This is a wonderfully simple way to harmonize body, mind and spirit. After a few minutes, continue breathing naturally but consider the exhalation to be the start of the breathing cycle, rather than the inhalation. Imagine the kind of labour that you would like to have. Visualize positions you will adopt, the way in which you will cope with contractions, whether you would like a therapist with you, the way the

cervix will open, the way your baby will descend down the birth canal. Above all, imagine it to be a positive experience.

THE HEART-UTERUS CONNECTION

The Chinese believe that, when a woman becomes pregnant, a direct channel of communication opens up between her heart and that of the baby. It is important that any concerns, fears and vulnerabilities that the mother has are dealt with. The strength of her heart and spirit helps to establish a strong bond with the baby. The acupoint that is used to strengthen this link is Heart 7, which is located on the inside of the wrist crease and has physical, mental and emotional significance. The Heart blood is regarded as the house of your spirit and the seat of all emotions. If your blood is low (that is, you are anaemic), you may become low in spirits, depressed and tearful. The Chinese also believe that *qi*, or life energy, which flows throughout the body, can be improved by focusing the mind, inducing a state of deep relaxation and encouraging positive thought.

THE VALUE OF YOGA

Yoga uses postures and breathing techniques to improve physical health and mental well-being (see page 142). It is important to strengthen the Heart *chakra* prior to labour, so that you are emotionally strong and you feel able to

cope with anything, rather than being nervous and vulnerable. There are techniques, drawing on these similar traditional beliefs, that can be used to prepare you mentally in the run-up to labour.

• Sit cross-legged on the floor. Rub your hands vigorously against your thighs to create heat in the palms. Place the right palm over the lower abdomen, covered by the left hand. Imagine that the baby is

ALTERNATE NOSTRIL BREATHING
This deep-breathing technique can be used to induce a state of calm (see also page 66).

lying beneath your hands. Slide your right hand out and place it, palm down, on the sacrum (at the back of the pelvis), with the left hand still in place.

• Alternatively, slide the back of both wrists up and down the kidney area of the lower back to help to prepare for delivery of the baby.

Natural Pain Relief

MANY WOMEN PREFER NOT TO USE DRUGS to deal with the pain of labour. If you are expecting your first baby, you may not know how much pain you can tolerate. Knowledge of various methods of pain relief will give you confidence and help you to develop a positive attitude to pain as a means of getting the baby born.

EFFECTS OF FEAR

It is important to appreciate the effects of fear on your labour. If you are frightened and in pain, the body releases the hormone adrenaline, producing the "fight or flight" response. Your circulatory, respiratory, genito-urinary, gastrointestinal and skeletal systems are all affected, resulting in increased blood sugar levels and heart rate, raised blood pressure and slower digestion. You will become agitated, the pain will increase and the progress of labour will be slowed. You should aim to feel as comfortable and secure as possible, happy in your environment and with the people who are supporting you.

THE BODY'S RESPONSE

The release of oxytocin shapes your contractions during labour. The hormone is produced as a result of pressure from the baby's head on the cervix: the greater the pressure, the more regular and consistent the contractions. Endorphins

are natural substances released by the body under stress. They have three main purposes: to modify pain, alter perception of time and space, and encourage well-being. Once labour begins, endorphin levels rise to help you to cope with painful contractions. If you are fearful, adrenaline will inhibit oxytocin and endorphin production.

NATURAL PAIN RELIEF

There are natural methods of pain relief that can be used as alternatives to conventional means such as anaesthetics

(for example, an epidural), inhaled analgesics (gas and air) or narcotics (pethidine).

• **Acupuncture** A qualified practitioner can help to relieve pain, boost energy levels and encourage you to control fear. Needles inserted into acupoints in the ear can be attached to an electro-acupuncture, or acutens, machine to stimulate the release of endorphins. You control the level of stimulation. You will feel a warm thudding sensation in your ear. It takes 30–40 minutes to build up the endorphin level enough to ease

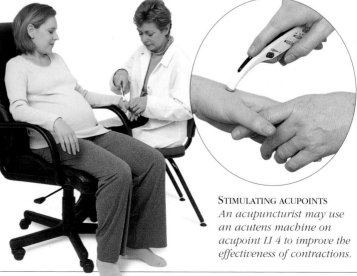

STIMULATING ACUPOINTS
An acupuncturist may use an acutens machine on acupoint LI 4 to improve the effectiveness of contractions.

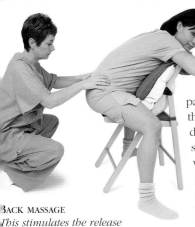

BACK MASSAGE
This stimulates the release of endorphins, the body's natural pain-killers.

painful contractions. To relieve backache, an acupuncturist will insert needles into acupoints Bl 31 and Bl 32 in the sacral region of the lower spine, or your partner can apply pressure. A TENS machine (*see page 109*) can also be used. This blocks pain receptors and is useful in early labour. Abdominal pain may be eased by treating acupoints Liv 3 (between the first and second toes) and GB 34 (outside leg just below the knee) to relax muscles and tendons. Acupuncture can also be used to improve weak or slow contractions by boosting the flow of *qi*. Again, Bl 31 and Bl 32 are the acupoints used.

• **Homeopathy** Remedies for pain relief include *Aconite 6c*, for contractions that occur in rapid succession with acute back pain; *Pulsatilla 6c*, for backache that is cutting and spasmodic; and *Belladonna 6c*, when pain extends from the back down the thighs. For abdominal pain try *Chamomilla 6c*, for spasmodic pain; and *Gelsemium 6c*, for cramps.

• **Massage** This is one of the simplest and most time-honoured ways of relieving pain. It helps to decrease the intensity of pain by dissipating tension. Massage should be rhythmical but varied, using different pressures and speeds. In general, a slow massage will calm and a brisk one will stimulate. Firm but gentle strokes using the flat of the hand and stroking towards the heart will ease tension. This should be done for at least 20 minutes to encourage endorphins to be released. Using the appropriate essential oil may be beneficial: lavender for relief of pain; mandarin to lift the spirits; and clary sage to improve contractions in an attempt to speed up a painful, protracted labour. Clary sage is a potent oil, however, and should

be pre-prepared by and used under strict instruction of a practitioner. Other suitable oils include chamomile, eucalyptus and frankincense.

OTHER USEFUL THERAPIES

• **Reflexology** Reflex points on the ankle bones correspond to the uterus and pelvic region. These can be stimulated in order to relieve pain and stress and to regulate contractions.
• **Hypnosis** Techniques of self-hypnosis to help you to control pain can be learnt beforehand.
• **Yoga** Regular yoga practice will put you in tune with your body so that you understand its natural responses during labour rather than resisting them and possibly losing control.

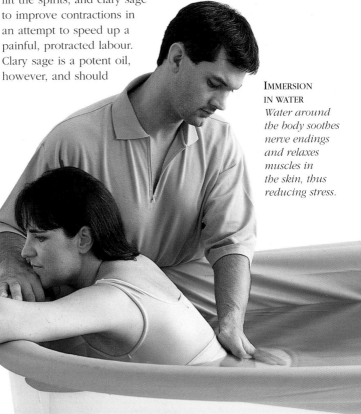

IMMERSION IN WATER
Water around the body soothes nerve endings and relaxes muscles in the skin, thus reducing stress.

Getting Ready to Go

As well as organizing the practical necessities for yourself during the birth, and for you and the baby afterwards, such as clothes, nappies and a camera, it is important to assemble items that will improve your general comfort as well as the remedies you have chosen to use to ease your way during labour.

BASIC NEEDS

At an antenatal clinic you will be given a list of items that you are recommended to take with you for the birth of your baby, including what is or is not provided by the hospital. In addition, consider the following.

• Socks and loose trousers. The Chinese tradition is to keep the feet and lower back warm in labour because of their link with the Kidney meridian.

• Snacks and drinks, including raspberry leaf tea.

• Distractions, such as magazines, playing cards and cassette tapes and a player, especially in early labour.

• General comfort aids, such as lipsalve, hair slides or bands, hand-held fan, tissues or wipes, face cloth or natural sponge, ice cubes, hot water bottle.

• TENS and acutens machines.

SOOTHING REMEDIES

Pick and choose complementary remedies from the following.

• **Aromatherapy massage oils** include: lavender, for anxiety; chamomile, clary sage (under direction), eucalyptus or lavender, for backache; clary sage, jasmine, lavender or rose, to stimulate contractions; frankincense or lavender for pain relief; lemon, lime and grapefruit, for refreshment; peppermint, for nausea.

• **Homeopathic remedies** *Arnica 6c*, taken before and after labour, for bruising; *Aconite 6c*, for shock and fear; *Caulophyllum 6c*, to induce or speed up contractions; *Pulsatilla 6c*, for emotional upset and changing moods; *Nux vomica 6c*, for nausea or backache.

• **Flower remedies** Cherry plum, if you have had enough; Five Flower Formula, for fear and panic; olive, in a lengthy labour; mugwort, in preparation for the final stage; and Rescue Remedy, for panic.

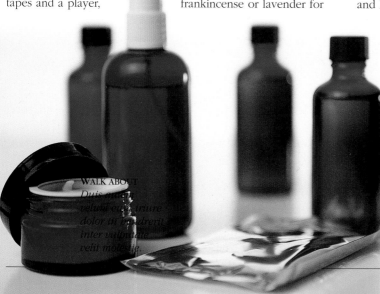

COMPLEMENTARY BIRTH KIT
You can buy ready-made kits of products for before, during and after the birth.
• *Preconditioning cream to prepare the nipples for breastfeeding.*
• *Preconditioning perineal oil to improve elasticity, thus reducing the risk of tearing.*
• *Labour massage oil to help to relieve discomfort.*
• *Energy drink specially formulated for labour.*
• *Facial spray to cool, refresh and revive.*

WALK ABOUT
Duis autem
velum eum iriure
dolor in hendrerit
inter vulputate
velit molestie.

Going into Labour

YOU MAY GO INTO LABOUR any time after 37 weeks of pregnancy. Do not worry that you might not realize you are going into labour when it starts. Although you may have been experiencing "practice" Braxton Hicks contractions for several weeks, there will be other signs that the birth is imminent.

RECOGNIZING THE SIGNS

There may be a combination of the following indications that labour has begun:
• **A show** This is a discharge of blood and mucus from the vagina up to a few days before or during the early first stage of labour. It occurs as the protective plug from the neck of the uterus is shed.
• **Waters leak or break** The bag of fluid surrounding the baby breaks, releasing its contents in a "flood" or, more commonly since the baby's head has probably engaged, in a trickle. Contact your midwife if this happens, even if you are not having contractions, because of the risk of infection.
• **Regular contractions** These may be felt initially as a constant, nagging backache, or you may have rhythmic, mildy painful contractions low in the back or abdomen.

WHAT TO DO

In the early stages of labour, as the cervix dilates the first 4 cm (1½ in), contractions will each last 50–60 seconds. They may still be inconsistent, but will probably be between five and ten minutes apart. Once your contractions seem regular, time them over an hour and note how long each one lasts. If you think you are in labour, phone your midwife or the hospital. Unless the contractions are very painful or every five minutes or more frequent, stay at home. You may be feeling excited, restless and nervous with anticipation. You will not feel like eating, drinking or sleeping. You will be able to move about as normal and be happy to have companionship, to talk and to be distracted.

USEFUL REMEDIES

How bearable the contractions are will depend on the baby's position (*see page 108*) and your own pain threshold. It is important to isolate and visualize exactly where the pain is in order to choose the most suitable remedy and make yourself more comfortable.
• Start using a TENS machine (*see page 109*), if you have one, to relieve back pain.

SOOTHING MASSAGE
Ask your partner to massage your lower back if you experience pain there in the early stage of labour.

• Apply gentle pressure to acupoints LI 4, sitiuated on the fleshy area at the base of the thumb and forefinger, or Sp 6, located in the middle of the inside leg four fingers' width above the ankle bone.
• Ask your partner or a friend to massage your back using lavender or rose essential oils.
• If you feel as if you are starting to panic, take Rescue Remedy, or if you feel afraid, mimulus flower remedy.

Inducing Labour

INDUCTION IS A DELIBERATE attempt to start labour by artificial means. Most women would prefer to go into labour naturally, but the safety of mother and baby is paramount. In certain circumstances the risk of continuing a pregnancy is greater than the potential risk of intervention by means of induction.

REASONS FOR INDUCTION

Rates of induction vary from hospital to hospital and from consultant to consultant. Find out what the induction policy is at your hospital so that you know what to expect if it is necessary. Induction may be recommended if:

• The baby has gone more than seven days beyond term (maximum 14 days). The danger is that the placenta will start to fail and the baby will lack oxygen. You may be asked to monitor the baby's activity.

• Your blood pressure is raised. Induction will depend upon the severity of your condition, the amount of protein in your urine and the maturity of the baby.

• You have gestational diabetes. This may put the baby at risk in late pregnancy. Induction may be recommended at about 37 weeks if there are indications that the baby is unwell.

• The membranes rupture early. Some hospitals advise induction, while others check that the umbilical cord has not come down and send you home to wait for labour to start.

• You have a poor obstetric history, for example placental abruption (placenta starts coming away from the uterine wall), stillbirth or foetal abnormality. A growing number of women want to know exactly when their baby will be born and request induction. It carries a risk, however, and should only be done for medical reasons.

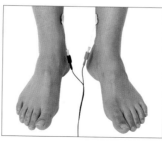

USING A **TENS** MACHINE
Attach a TENS machine (see page 109) to Sp 6 on each inside leg, four fingers' width above the ankle, to start induction.

METHODS OF INDUCTION

The following methods or products may be used.

• Sweeping the membranes. This can be done as part of a vaginal examination. It may be a little painful but can induce labour if you are close to term.

• Prostaglandin gel. Pessaries containing this hormone are inserted into the vagina, or gel is applied around the cervix (unless the membranes have ruptured), to ripen the cervix and stimulate contractions.

• Intravenous oxytocin. You will be put on a drip of this drug to initiate contractions.

NATURAL ALTERNATIVES

If labour begins spontaneously, contractions build up gradually. Endorphins are released to help you to cope with the build-up of pain. If you are induced, this natural process is short-circuited. The pain comes fast and can be acute. Without the chance to prepare, many women lose control and demand pain relief. You will usually be given several days' notice of an induction, which gives you the opportunity to try natural alternatives. Only do this if your pregnancy has been free of complications and you are at term. Consult your midwife first.

• **Acupuncture** Needles will be inserted into acupoints on the back. Two or three sessions over a week may be necessary. Also try acupressure or a TENS machine on LI 4 and Sp 6.

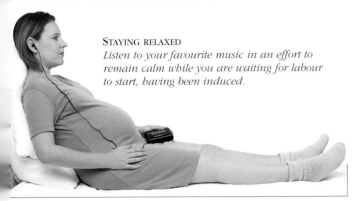

STAYING RELAXED
Listen to your favourite music in an effort to remain calm while you are waiting for labour to start, having been induced.

• **Homeopathy** Take *Secale 30c* or *Caulophyllum 30c* (as directed by a practitioner) until your contractions start. *Caulophyllum* should not be used if you have a history of quick labour.

• **Reflexology** Treatment will be applied to the pituitary reflexes. It is advisable to consult a qualified practitioner.

• **Cranial osteopathy** This may stimulate the pituitary gland to produce the hormones that are important for labour.

• **Herbalism** Drink raspberry leaf tea four times a day.

COPING WITH INDUCTION

Once labour is underway, you may well need some help in dealing with contractions.

• **Acupressure**. With advice from a practitioner beforehand, mark the relevant acupoints on your body and apply a TENS machine (*see page 109*) to stimulate them or get your partner to massage them if the pain is severe. Use Bl 31 and Bl 32 in the sacral region of the lower back for back pain and Sp 8 on the inside lower leg for abdominal pain. Alternatively, take an acupuncturist with you into the delivery room.

• **Flower remedies** A few drops directly on the tongue or added to a glass of water may help you to cope as labour progresses. Take Five Flower Formula or Rescue Remedy for panic, shock or fear; cherry plum if you are at the end of your tether; gorse if you feel hopeless and that your labour is endless; and rock rose for fear and panic.

• **Homeopathy** A homeopath may attend the birth or give advice over the phone, having prepared various remedies for you in advance. These might include *Aconite 6c*, for severe, rapid contractions, soreness in the back and fear; *Chamomilla 6c*, for

PROVIDING SUPPORT
Pain can come fast and strong. In this position a partner can provide support as well as reassurance.

unbearable, spasmodic contractions, back pain and oversensitivity to noise and pain; *Cimic. 6c*, for severe contractions, a bruised feeling, restlessness, irritability and chilliness; *Coffea 6c*, for severe back pain and the urge to bear down before the cervix is fully dilated; *Secale cornutum 6c*, for irregular, ineffectual contractions that are causing distress.

• **Aromatherapy** For backache, massage with lavender, clary sage (under direction by a practitioner) or chamomile oils diluted in a carrier oil; for encouraging contractions and labour, lavender, clary sage, jasmine or rose; to refresh and revitalize, a drop of lemon, lime or grapefruit placed in the palm of the hand; for hysteria, a drop of frankincense placed in the palm of the hand.

First Stage of Labour

ACQUAINTING YOURSELF WITH THE DIFFERENT STAGES and behaviour patterns of labour is useful preparation for the event and will help you greatly when the time comes, especially if you are apprehensive or even fearful. In addition, there is a wealth of gentle, complementary remedies to assist you in labour.

KEY TIPS

Maintain upright postitions as much as possible

✻

Rest between contractions

✻

Drink plenty of fluids

✻

Concentrate on breathing

WHAT HAPPENS

The length of the first stage of labour with a first baby is on average 12–14 hours (less in subsequent pregnancies). The cervix opens gradually, dilating to 10 cm at the rate of approximately 1 cm an hour. The baby moves down into the pelvis, gradually turning so that it is facing is your back.

THE ROLE OF YOUR MIDWIFE

A midwife's job is to keep an eye on both you and the baby, checking the progress of your labour. Initially she will palpate your abdomen gently to see how the baby is lying and how far the head is engaged. She will note your temperature, pulse rate, blood pressure and any swelling of the ankles. She will listen to the baby's heartbeat, which should be strong and regular (110–150 beats a minute). You may be attached to a cardiotachograph (CTG) machine, which monitors contractions and the baby's heartbeat. Every 4–5 hours your

midwife will give you a vaginal examination to assess how far the cervix has dilated.

THE BABY'S POSITION

The way the baby is lying at the end of your pregnancy will have a significant effect on the kind of labour you are likely to have. The most favourable position is with the baby's back facing your front: the occipital anterior position. Many babies today, especially with first-time mothers and often as a result of a sedentary lifestyle, present in the occipital posterior position, with the baby's back facing your back. The baby will turn

during delivery, but this may prolong your labour (*see page 109,* Coping with *Induction, for dealing with a difficult labour*). To help the baby get into position in the final weeks of pregnancy, avoid sitting cross-legged; stand leaning forward against a wall for 10–20 minutes twice a day in the last six weeks; avoid reclining positions, such as sitting slumped on a sofa; and go swimming and practise yoga, which are helpful forms of gentle exercise.

EARLY LABOUR

As the cervix dilates from 0 cm to 4 cm try to conserve energy but keep mobile, using gravity to help the baby's head to descend and press on the cervix, keeping contractions going. If necessary, squat or sit on a chair during contractions. If you

TAKING UP POSITIONS
Your midwife will help you to relax into positions that help your labour to progress and ensure that you breathe correctly.

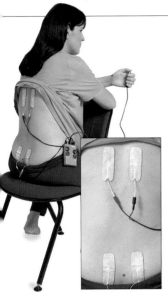

TENS MACHINE
*Pads are easily attached to
specific points on the back
to block pain messages.*

have back pain, kneel on
all fours and ask your partner
to massage your back. This
position will help the pelvis
to open: also try rocking the
pelvis. Develop your own
pattern of breathing, slowly to
keep calm, faster as the body
requires more oxygen.

ACCELERATED PHASE

Once labour is established,
the contractions will speed up,
occurring every 2–3 minutes,
lasting 45–60 seconds, and
feeling stronger and more
intense. During this phase,
your cervix will dilate from
4 cm to 8 cm. This is a good
time to get into a birthing pool
or bath. You will want to rest
between contractions by now,
finding the most comfortable
position and supported by your
partner or midwife and by
pillows and cushions. It may be
difficult to get comfortable and
your partner's support will be

vitally important. You will have
lost your appetite but you will
be thirsty. You may become
withdrawn, avoiding eye contact
and conversation. Your partner
should be aware that you will
not want noise or disruption.
Try the following remedies
and methods of pain relief.
• Use a TENS (Transcutaneous
Electrical Nerve Stimulation)
machine (*see left*). Electrodes
in pads are attached to specific
points on the back. A pulsed
electric current blocks pain
messages from the cervix and
uterus to the brain. A control
box allows you to alter the
intensity of the current. A TENS
machine can be bought or hired
a few weeks before the birth.
• Try to identify the location
of pain and the nature of other
problems, such as slow or
ineffectual contractions, and
use the appropriate remedies
(*see pages 102–3*).
• Take Rescue Remedy or
mimulus flower remedy if you
are feeling fearful or panicky.
• Use essential oils of lavender,
frankincense, mandarin and
chamomile to help to relieve
anxiety or stress. Massage a
drop of whichever you like
into the plam of your hand
to release the aroma.
• If you feel nauseous, sniff
peppermint essential oil.
• Take *Pulsatilla 6c* (dosage:
every 20 minutes for up to
seven doses) if you feel weepy,
you keep apologising and your
mood is very changeable.
• Try to maintain positions that
help to tilt your pelvis forward
and encourage the baby into
the most desirable position for
the birth, open up the pelvic

outlet and keep contractions
going (*see opposite, below and
see also pages 74–5*).

TRANSITION

This is often the most difficult
part of labour, as the cervix
dilates to 10 cm (4 in) and
the opening out phase changes
to the bearing down phase.
Contractions will be at their
strongest, 1–3½ minutes
apart and lasting 45–90
seconds. It will be
hard to stay in
control: you may
feel nauseous,
shivery, irritable
and anxious. Take
Rescue Remedy and
star of Bethlehem
flower remedy
if you are
struggling. Some
women prefer
to get out of a
birthing pool
at this stage.

**KEEPING
UPRIGHT**
*Encourage the
baby's head to
descend and
keep contractions
going by being
upright. Rest
by leaning
against a wall
for support with
knees bent slightly.*

Second Stage of Labour

THE SECOND STAGE OF LABOUR is the period from full dilation of the cervix to the birth. On average, this lasts about an hour in a first pregnancy but less in subsequent ones. With a renewed burst of energy, you will develop a strong and irresistible urge to push the baby down the birth canal.

HOW YOU WILL FEEL

The transition phase brings a surge of endorphins before the urge to push signals the start of the second stage. You may feel calmer, with a renewed sense of focus and purpose. You will begin to feel more passive, less active. Find a position that is comfortable. Try squatting, supported by your partner, on all fours or over a bean bag, or kneeling on a bed. Once the cervix is fully dilated, the pain feels like cramp or a burning sensation. Contractions will be shorter and further apart. Your waters will break if they have not already done so. The urge to push builds gradually. Follow this urge as it suits you: do what your body feels it has to.

USING REMEDIES

Complentary remedies may be useful in the second stage.
• Apply gentle pressure to acupoints GB 21, at the top of the shoulder near the neck, or LI 4, between the forefinger and thumb to stimulate contractions if they are infrequent or the gap between them lengthens.

KNEELING ON ALL FOURS
Kneeling may be less tiring than other positions. Keep your back straight and relax forwards on to a cushion between contractions.

• Homeopathic remedies include: *Coffea 6c* if you are despairing, with no urge to push; *Kali carb. 6c* if you have become obstinate and dilation has ceased; *Secale 6c* if you are distressed and want to push.
• Mugwort flower remedy promotes birthing, five flower formula will help you stay calm and centred and walnut may help you to adjust to the rapid physical changes.
• Essential oils of lemon, lime, grapefruit, mandarin, jasmine or rose – vapourized or used for gentle massage – will lift mood.

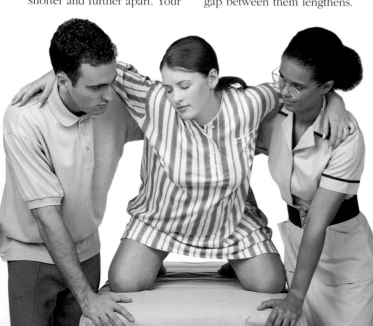

POSITION FOR DELIVERY
Kneeling is a good position from which to push. Your midwife and partner can support you.

Third Stage of Labour

THE THIRD STAGE OF LABOUR follows the birth and lasts about 30 minutes. During this time the "afterbirth" (placenta and membranes) is delivered, but you will be concentrating on your new baby. You may well be feeling euphoric, with a strong urge to bond as you hold your baby to your breast.

KEY TIPS

Talk to your midwife about active management before the birth

❊

Keep warm and out of draughts

❊

Spend time quietly alone with your partner and baby as soon as possible after the birth

THE BIRTH

As the baby is born, your midwife will control its passage through the vagina so as to minimize the risk of tearing the perineum. Once the head has been born, the shoulders and the rest of the body quickly follow and your baby is delivered on to your stomach. As the baby's shoulder is presented, you may be given an injection of a drug called syntometrine. This makes the womb contract and expel the placenta quickly, thus preventing excessive bleeding. This is known as active management of the third stage. It does carry a small risk of minor side effects to you and the baby. Discuss with your midwife whether or not you want this. Your attention will by now, however, be entirely focused on your new baby, and you will have few memories of the physical sensations of the third stage. Endorphins released during the birth promote a euphoric state and strengthen the natural urge to bond. You may feel elated, with a strong instinct to sit up and gather your baby to the breast.

USING NATURAL REMEDIES

These can be used for several purposes after the birth.
• For a retained placenta, apply pressure to acupoints CV 4 on the lower abdomen, Bl 67 on the little toe nail, or GB 21 in the shoulder "well". Alternatively, massage the abdomen with diluted clary sage oil, take

the homeopathic remedy *Caulophyllum 6c* or mugwort flower remedy to encourage uterine contractions.
• To relieve after pains, shock, soft-tissue damage, soreness, swelling and bruising, take *Arnica 6c*. Also for shock, try *Aconite 6c* or Rescue Remedy or Five Flower Formula.

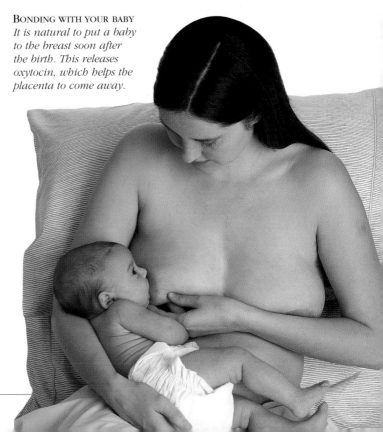

BONDING WITH YOUR BABY
It is natural to put a baby to the breast soon after the birth. This releases oxytocin, which helps the placenta to come away.

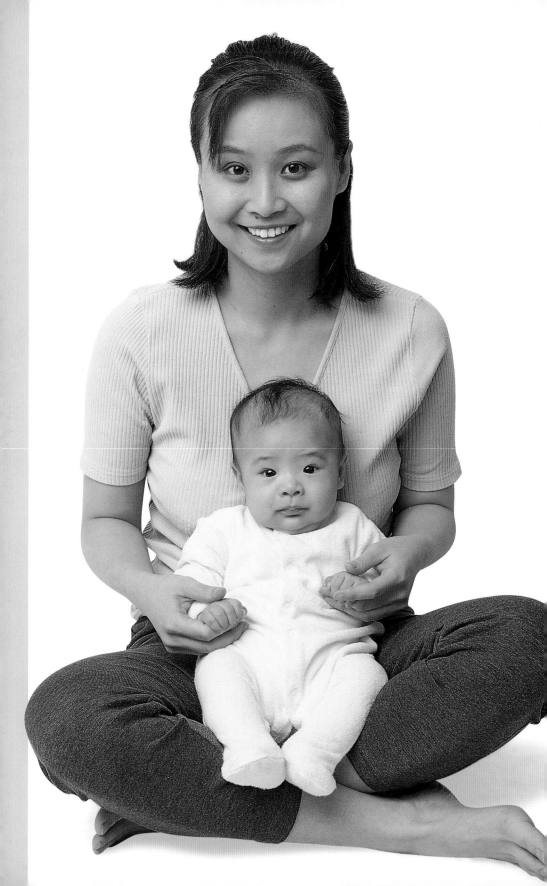

THE FIRST DAYS AND WEEKS after giving birth to your baby are known as the fourth trimester or puerperium – the period belonging to the child. It is the time during which your reproductive organs return to their pre-pregnant state and, more importantly, the time in which you start to adjust to the presence of a new person in

The postnatal period

your life and in your family. This chapter takes you through the day-by-day changes of the early postnatal period, offering advice on nutrition, exercise and ways of helping your body to heal quickly. It also gives practical self-help solutions to some of the problems that you may encounter, such as difficulties with breastfeeding.

DAY-BY-DAY DEVELOPMENTS

ONCE YOU'VE GIVEN BIRTH, you will probably feel elated, excited and relieved. Your body will go through great changes in the next few days. Do not underestimate the adjustments you will have to make on every level now that you are a mother.

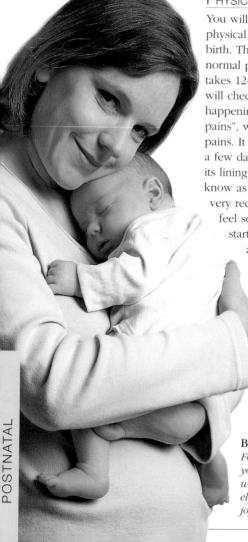

PHYSICAL CHANGES

You will experience noticeable physical changes following the birth. The uterus returns to its normal position; this usually takes 12–15 days. Your midwife will check daily that this is happening. You may get "after pains", which resemble period pains. It is normal to bleed for a few days as the uterus sheds its lining. This discharge is know as lochea and is initially very red. Your perineum may feel sore and bruised, but start pelvic floor exercises as soon as you can. Your blood volume will decrease and you may pass more urine than usual. At first the breasts produce colostrum. Whether or not you have decided to breastfeed, milk will flood in on day

BUNDLE OF JOY
Following the birth of your baby your emotions will include excitement, elation, pride, wonder, joy and profound relief.

three. On an emotional level, happiness may be tempered by anxiety about the baby and your new responsibilities. Add to that exhaustion and physical discomfort and you have the ingredients for a volatile emotional cocktail.

DOING THINGS

If you are home by day three or four, it is especially important that you do not overdo it. Take the phone off the hook, limit the number of visitors and make the most of your time with your partner and new baby. You may feel daunted without the support of a midwife, but you will soon get used to caring for your baby's needs. Be prepared for disrupted nights. The "baby blues" may arrive on days three to five; 70–80 per cent of new mothers are affected. Find time to relax and rest frequently. Try to get out for a walk by day six. By the end of the first week, any stitches should be healing, soreness disappearing, nipples getting used to feeding and you and your baby will be getting to know each other very well.

POSTNATAL

THE FIRST WEEK

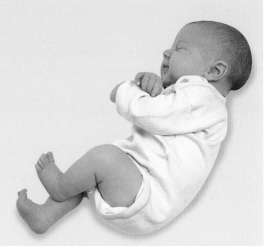

DAY 1: Soon after the birth, simple tests will be carried out to see if your baby is healthy. Pink skin indicates good respiration; the pulse reveals strength and regularity of heartbeat; facial expressions and crying show alertness; movement indicates healthy muscles; and good breathing means healthy lungs. The midwife also checks the baby's facial features, body proportions, spine, legs, fingers and toes and anus. She measures the circumference of the head and length of body, weighs the baby and takes its temperature.

DAY 2: More thorough tests are done: the head and neck are checked for misshaping and abnormality; the heart and lungs are listened to; arms and hands are examined for strength and movement; the abdomen is palpated to check the liver and spleen; genitals are looked over; hips, legs and feet are moved to detect dislocation, length and size and the health of nerves and muscles.

DAY 3: At first a baby receives colostrum, which provides water, protein, sugar, vitamins, minerals and antibodies. Between three and five days after the birth, milk production begins. A baby digests a full feed of breast milk in 1½–2 hours, after which it demands more. Research shows that fed-on-demand babies gain weight quicker than those fed every 3–4 hours.

DAY 4: A newborn baby appears fragile but is in fact quite resilient. It does, however, thrive on being nursed and cuddled frequently, especially with skin-to-skin contact, which stimulates its senses of touch and smell. Research suggests that the more physical contact a baby has, the happier and healthier it becomes. A baby will cry if it feels abandoned and lonely. It likes to be handled firmly and confidently, and will need its head supported for several weeks.

DAY 5: A newborn's senses of hearing, sight, smell and taste are fairly well developed. Your baby will soon recognize you by smell and by sight within a couple of weeks. If held close, the baby will focus on your face. It has certain reflexes from birth: its fingers will grasp anything placed in its palm; it can make stepping movements; if its cheek is stroked, it will turn its head, or root, to find the nipple; and, if startled, it will throw its arms and legs out – which is known as the Moro reflex. All babies also have sucking and swallowing reflexes.

DAY 6: Your baby can communicate from birth. Crying is the most obvious way of signalling and there are different kinds of cries depending on whether the baby is hungry, lonely, uncomfortable or tired. A baby will respond to its parents' voices and faces by moving its mouth rather like a fish feeding, perhaps sticking its tongue out, changing its breathing or jerking its limbs.

DAY 7: On day six or seven your baby will be given a Guthrie test. A drop of blood is taken from the heel to check the functioning of the thyroid and for a rare disorder that causes mental retardation (phenylketonuria). Your baby may sleep for up to 16 hours a day but will have no concept as yet of night and day.

POSTNATAL

Nutrition for Mother & Baby

MAINTAINING A HIGHLY NUTRITIOUS DIET after the birth is equally as important as it was during your pregnancy because many extra demands continue to be made on your body. If you are breastfeeding, your diet needs to supply a variety of key nutrients for the baby and to speed your recovery from the birth.

KEY TIPS

Plan meals in advance to save time and ensure a balanced diet

✻

Drink plenty of fluids if you are breastfeeding

✻

Continue to include plenty of "brain foods" in your diet

THE FIRST FEW WEEKS

The weeks following the birth of your baby can be a stressful time. If you had a Caesarean section delivery, you will be recovering; if you had an episiotomy, the perineum will be healing. Your nights are bound to be disturbed by the baby's feeding regime, so you will be feeling tired. You will also be adjusting to your additional responsibilities and the fact that the family has a new member. All in all, you may well have difficulty finding the time to prepare nourishing meals. During the last few weeks of your pregnancy it is well worth planning a nutrition programme for two weeks after the birth and, if possible, preparing and freezing some simple yet nutritious meals.

BENEFITS OF BREAST MILK

Breast milk contains proteins, carbohydrates, essential fatty acids, minerals, salts, enzymes, vitamins and hormones, all in perfect proportion to suit the infant digestive system. A mother's milk is also full of antibodies to help the baby's immature immune system and provide protection against allergies. Colostrum, the breast milk produced during the first three days after birth, is the best food that your baby can have. Breastfed babies seem to suffer less from conditions such as schizophrenia and ADHD (attention deficit hyperactivity disorder). They appear to maintain better intellectual ability in later life, almost certainly because breast milk contains plenty of essential fatty acids – vital for brain growth in the first few months after birth.

KEY NUTRIENTS

If you are breastfeeding, you should drink plenty of water, since you lose up to 700 ml (1¼ pints) of fluid a day. You should also make sure that you maintain supplies of

KEY DAILY DIETARY CONSTITUENTS

7 serving of grains
6 servings of vegetables
4 servings of fruit, 2 of which are rich in vitamin C
3 servings of lean meat
3 servings of calcium-rich food
1 serving of magnesium-rich food

AVOCADO SALAD
Avocado teamed with parma ham, pink grapefruit, and rocket in a honey and poppy seed dressing provides a tasty, nutrient-filled brunch.

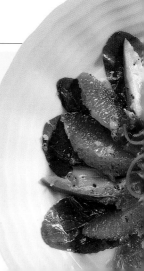

certain essential nutrients for yourself and for the baby.

• Vitamin A, to strengthen the baby's immune system and the development of vision, hearing and taste. Sources: apricots, carrots, spinach, broccoli, oily fish, eggs, butter, cheese.

• B vitamins, for lactation and to help to prevent fluctuations in blood sugar levels. Sources: meat, poultry, vegetables, eggs, milk, pulses, nuts, wholegrains. B vitamins include folate, for red blood cell formation and for brain and nerve function. Sources: broccoli, spinach, wheatgerm, seeds, nuts.

• Vitamin C, for making blood vessels, collagen and connective tissue necessary for wound healing, for strengthening the immune system and improving iron absorption. Sources: citrus fruits, blackcurrants, tomatoes, peppers, dark green vegetables.

• Vitamin D, to aid calcium absorption, thus maintaining healthy bones. Sources: milk, eggs, oily fish, brown rice.

• Vitamin E, for anti-oxidant protection, neural development and the healing of wounds. Sources: avocado, nuts, seeds, olives, blackberries, brown rice.

•Vitamin K, for blood clotting. The baby cannot yet make vitamin K for itself, so still relies on you for its supply. Sources: green leafy vegetables, cauliflower, avocado.

• Calcium, to replenish that supplied to the baby in breast milk. Sources: yogurt, milk, nuts, pulses, wholegrains.

• Iron, for the manufacture of haemoglobin and for fighting infection. This is particularly important if you lost blood during the birth. Sources: meat, poultry, dark oily fish, dried fruit, green leafy vegetables.

• Zinc, for wound healing, hormone production and to help to prevent postnatal depression. Levels of copper, which reduces the effectiveness of zinc, rise during pregnancy, reaching a peak immediately after the birth. Unless you boost your zinc levels, it is likely that both you and the baby will be zinc deficient. (The placenta is an exceedingly rich source of zinc, which is why most animals eat theirs).

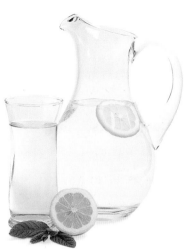

WATER SUPPLIES
Drink plenty of fresh water throughout the day if you are breastfeeding in order to replenish lost fluids.

Sources: red meat, poultry, seafood, eggs, cheese, peanuts.

• DHA (docosahexaenoic acid), an essential fatty acid that is vitally important for the development of a baby's brain. Breast-fed babies have higher levels of DHA than bottle-fed babies. However, levels of DHA in breast milk have fallen by 35 per cent in the last 15 years as general consumption of oily fish has decreased for a number of reasons.

SUGGESTED MEAL PLAN

BREAKFAST
Muesli with milk, sunflower seeds, Brazil nuts, wheatgerm and apricots

MIDMORNING SNACK
Oatcakes and sardines

LUNCH
Wholewheat pasta with cheese and spinach sauce; tropical fruit salad with mango and papaya

AFTERNOON SNACK
Yogurt with banana, wheatgerm and sesame seeds

DINNER
Chicken and chickpea stew with peppers, peas and sweet potatoes

BEDTIME SNACK
Wholemeal bread and butter

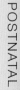

POSTNATAL

Postnatal Exercise

EVEN WHILE STILL PREGNANT, MANY WOMEN ASK how soon after the birth they can exercise again. The answer depends upon how you feel and what type of birth you had: how long and tiring it was; or whether or not you had stitches, for example. Give your body time to recover before you begin strenuous exercise.

GENERAL GUIDELINES

You should still, following the birth, be aware of the general guidelines relating to exercise during pregnancy (*see pages 18–19*). It is very important to warm up before doing any form of exercise and to cool down when you have finished (*see pages 32*). Once the baby has been delivered, your uterus will start to shrink back to its pre-pregnant state, but at first your abdomen will feel slack. You may wonder if you will ever have a waist or a flat stomach again. The good news is that you can start doing gentle exercises as soon as you feel fit enough. Do not forget pelvic floor exercises (*see page 75*).

EARLY ABDOMINALS

Exercises to tone the stomach muscles are obviously high on every woman's list of priorities for postnatal exercising. Following a normal delivery a midwife will examine your abdomen to check that the uterus is shrinking back, and she will be able to judge how well everything is returning to normal. As long as she is satisfied that it is, you can start doing pelvic tilts, or static abdominal contractions, (*see pages 50–1*) while you are still in hospital. These are a good means of getting tone back and you can do them every day – sitting down, standing up or on all fours. If you have had

a Caesarean section (*see pages 126–7*), you will be encouraged to get out of bed quite soon, and you, too, can start to do these abdominal exercises very gently. Always be guided by your midwife or an obstetric physiotherapist, however. If your wound is slow to heal or if you have an infection, you should not exercise.

LATER ABDOMINALS

Consult your midwife or an exercise teacher about doing more strenuous abdominal exercises. This is not advisable until the gap between the muscle halves of the rectus abdominis (part of the corset of abdominal muscles) is less than

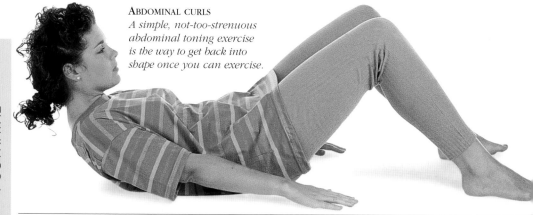

ABDOMINAL CURLS
A simple, not-too-strenuous abdominal toning exercise is the way to get back into shape once you can exercise.

POSTNATAL

DIAGONAL REACHES

*L*IE ON YOUR BACK WITH KNEES BENT, *feet flat on the floor and arms by your sides. Pull in the abdominal muscles and tilt the pelvis upwards. Lift your head and shoulders off the floor and reach your left hand across to your right ankle. Slowly lower yourself back on to the floor and relax your abdomen. Repeat, reaching the right hand to the left ankle. Repeat the sequence ten times.*

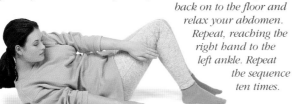

two fingers' width apart. Then you can begin to do sit-ups (abdominal curls).

• **Abdominal curls** (*see opposite*) Lie on your back (with a pillow under your head if you prefer), with knees bent, feet flat on the floor, and hands by your sides. Pull in the abdominal muscles, tighten the muscles in the buttocks and tilt the pelvis upwards. Pressing the small of the back into the floor, lift the head and shoulders off the floor. Exhale as you lift up and inhale as you lower back down. Repeat ten times. Then do the same number of diagonal reaches (*see above*), breathing out as you lift up and in as you lower back down.

EXERCISING OTHER PARTS

Your postnatal exercise programme should include exercises that tone up other parts of the body, such as the waist and the legs; help to prevent physical problems, such as poor circulation (*see page 51*); and increase your stamina so that you can cope with the demands of looking after a small baby. Toning exercises might include leg lifts

(*see below*) and box-position press-ups. Build up stamina levels by doing the same aerobic exercises as you did antenatally (*see page 33*), but gradually increasing the number of repeats and the amount of effort you put in until you are ready to return to your pre-pregnancy exercise programme.

• **Box-position press-ups** Kneel on the floor, with knees

directly under the hips and hands directly under the shoulders, fingers pointing forwards. Breathe in as you bend the elbows, taking the chin and chest towards the floor between the hands. Keep the back flat. Straighten the arms as you breathe out. Repeat eight times.

RETURNING TO NORMAL

Resuming the exercise regime that you had before pregnancy will depend on many things, not least of which are your physical condition and the time you have available. Do not exercise if you are tired, and remember that, if you do not have time to attend an exercise class, pushing a pram for half an hour is itself good exercise. Build up your fitness gradually and discuss your readiness at your last postnatal check-up.

LEG LIFTS

1 *L*IE ON YOUR SIDE *with the legs out in a straight line, one arm supporting the head, and the other on the floor in front of you for balance.*

2 *R*AISE THE TOP LEG SLOWLY *and smoothly and lower. Repeat 5–10 times, then turn on to your other side and repeat with the other leg.*

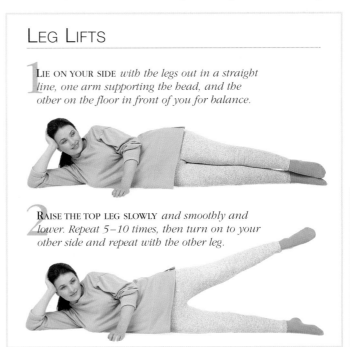

POSTNATAL

Five-point Action Plan

IN MEDICAL TERMS, the first few days and weeks after the birth of your baby are called the puerperium, which is defined as the period in which your reproductive organs return to their pre-pregnant state. It is also, more importantly, the time when you begin to adjust to a new person in your life. The following tips might be helpful.

ENJOY THE EXPERIENCE

Laughter and tears, excitement and anxiety, elation and exhaustion, a huge sense of achievement and an overwhelming feeling of responsibility: you will be feeling all this and more, with one emotion quickly following another. This roller-coaster of emotion is normal, so try to enjoy the ride and make the most of the first few days with your new baby before the rest of the world and everyday life intrude.

REST & RECUPERATE

Your body is once again going through enormous changes and it needs a renewal period for recovery and healing. Sleep when your baby sleeps and give your body the best chance for regeneration. Remember that tiredness will affect milk production if you are breastfeeding. Take gentle remedies and use natural products to ease conditions arising from the birth of your baby – from soreness to shock.

DELAY RETURNING TO NORMAL

Do not try to overachieve and accept any help you are offered, whether it is to cook a meal, do the shopping or take older children off your hands for a few hours. Keep your pyjamas on for as long as possible when you come home from hospital, because as soon as you get dressed you will be tempted to "resume normal service". It is worth remembering that in eastern cultures, women are expected to rest for 40 days after giving birth to a child.

FOLLOW YOUR INSTINCTS

The early days with a new baby can be fraught, especially if it is your first and you are concerned about not knowing what to do. Trust your instincts and try not to be confused by conflicting advice from well-meaning family and friends. It may be helpful to consult a friend who has older children and whose judgment you respect. Do not be reluctant to share any concerns with your midwife or health visitor.

EAT WELL

Good nutrition, as always, is vitally important, especially if you are breastfeeding. Of particular significance are zinc, for the production of hormones and to help to combat postnatal depression, and vitamin C, to help to fight infection, heal any wounds, and assist in the absorption of iron. Remember to maintain a good fluid intake, preferably water, herbal teas or diluted fruit juices.

POSTNATAL

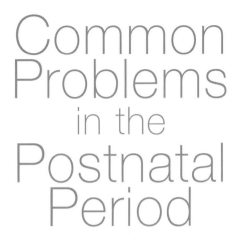

Common Problems in the Postnatal Period

So, YOUR BABY HAS BEEN BORN, with all the excitement that such a momentous event brings. Now you must look after yourself, as well as you do the baby. You need to recover from the birth and enjoy your new situation, using gentle treatments to soothe away any postnatal problems.

POSTNATAL

Breastfeeding Problems

THE ANTIBODIES IN BREAST MILK are your baby's main protection against disease and allergy. In addition, colostrum, the thick, nutrient-rich fluid produced in the first few days after the birth, is easily absorbed into the baby's bloodstream and protects and lines the gut. Breastfeeding is therefore to be recommended, but problems may arise in the beginning.

POSSIBLE PROBLEMS

Sore or cracked nipples

Engorgement

Insufficient lactation

Blocked ducts and mastitis

AROMATHERAPY

Soothing oils can help to relieve **engorgement** and **mastitis**. The former occurs when the breasts are overfilled with milk, making them swollen and uncomfortable Continue to feed your baby and the soreness and swelling should subside within 24–36 hours. Mastitis, which can cause engorgement, may result from a blocked duct or infection entering the nipple. It requires conventional treatment but the following may help to relieve discomfort.

* To reduce **engorgement**, place a few drops of jasmine oil on to some cotton wool and inhale.
* If you have **mastitis**, soak your feet every two hours in a warm foot bath containing a few drops of eucalyptus oil to help to ease your general discomfort.

Caution: use essential oils sparingly near your body in order not to overload the baby's olfactory system; see page 153 for oils to avoid.

See page 152–3 for further information

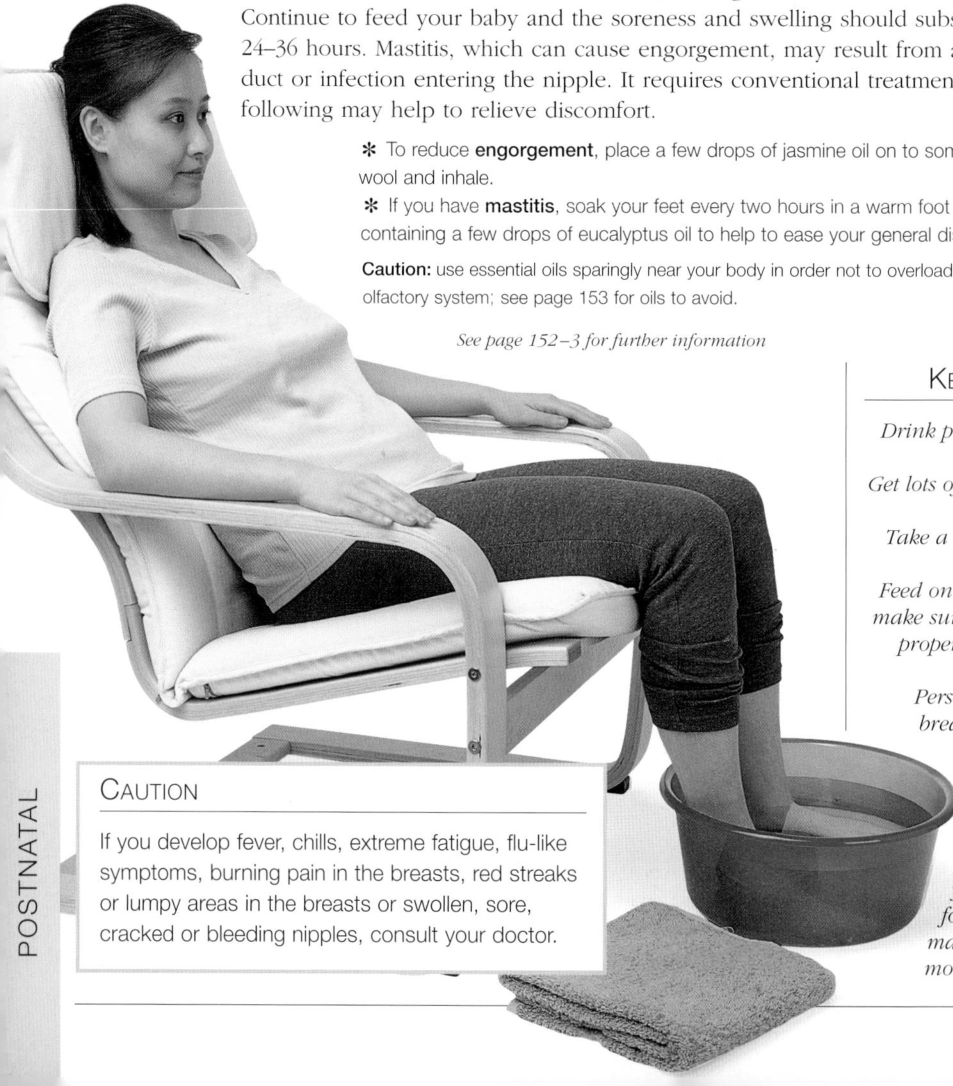

KEY TIPS

Drink plenty of water

Get lots of sleep and rest

Take a multivitamin

Feed on demand and make sure your baby is properly attached

Persevere with breastfeeding

RELIEVING DISCOMFORT *Relaxing while soaking your feet in a foot bath will make you feel more comfortable.*

CAUTION

If you develop fever, chills, extreme fatigue, flu-like symptoms, burning pain in the breasts, red streaks or lumpy areas in the breasts or swollen, sore, cracked or bleeding nipples, consult your doctor.

COMPLEMENTARY TREATMENTS

Before using a complementary treatment, please read any **Cautions** and the relevant page references

PRACTICAL MEASURES as well as complementary treatments can help to prevent or solve many breastfeeding problems. Some problems are due to poor feeding techniques. Support your back with pillows and lift the baby to your breast rather than bending over it. Place a cushion beneath the baby if it helps. Eat between 2,200 and 2,700 calories a day while you are breastfeeding. You need to include several portions a day of calcium-rich foods, fruits and vegetables, grains and meat, fish or poultry in your diet. You should also make sure that you eat rich food sources of zinc, selenium and vitamins E and K. Take a fish-oil supplement while breastfeeding if you are deficient in fatty acids.

ACUPUNCTURE

Insufficient lactation may be improved by acupuncture. Breast milk usually arrives on the third day after the birth, but it may be later following a Caesarean section. Anaemia, anxiety and exhaustion all reduce milk production. Rest and keep feeding. Avoid using nipple shields.

✳ Acupuncture, acupressure or shiatsu on SI1, on the nail point of the little finger, and CV17, between the breasts, can both help to stimulate milk production.

See page 134–5 for further information

HOMEOPATHY

Homeopathic remedies may be of help for breastfeeding problems. **Sore or cracked nipples** are common and often caused by the baby not latching on properly. Avoid frequent washing and dry well. After a feed, wipe some milk around each nipple and let them dry naturally. Expose them to the air freqently.

✳ For **sore or cracked nipples** that are bleeding or swollen, *Graphites 6c*; for cracked nipples, *Staphysagria 6c*; for cracked, bleeding, stinging, burning or itching nipples, *Lycopodium 6c*; and for sore nipples accompanied by tearfulness and timidity, *Pulsatilla 6c*.

BELLADONNA
This has long been prescribed for fever and inflammation.

✳ For **engorgement** with hard, hot, inflamed and throbbing breasts, *Belladonna 6c*; for hard,hot and pale breasts with stitching pains, *Bryonia 6c*.

✳ For **insufficient lactation**, when milk is slow to come in, *Urtica urens 6c*; if milk flow ceases, *Agnus 6c*.

✳ For **mastitis** with hot, red and inflamed breasts and a fever, *Belladonna 30c*; for a suspected breast abscess or mastitis, *Bryonia 30c*; for red, inflamed and itchy breasts, *Sulphur 6c*.

See page 148–9 for further information

WESTERN HERBALISM

A blocked milk duct, often caused by pressure from tight clothing or incorrect positioning of the baby, appears as a red patch. It may lead to bacterial infection (mastitis). Consult your doctor in case an abscess develops. Apply hot flannels and massage the area.

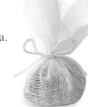

✳ For **mastitis**, apply a poultice of slippery elm, cooked bran or linseed. Drink yarrow or elderflower tea if you have a fever.

✳ For **engorgement**, place cabbage leaves (preferably dark green) on the affected area inside your bra.

CHAMOMILE TEA
Place used tea bags directly on to the nipples to relieve soreness.

✳ For **sore or cracked nipples**, put grated raw carrot or potato directly on to the nipple or steep two chamomile tea bags in boiling water and, when cooled, place over the nipples inside your bra (protect clothing from staining). Apply calendula, chamomile or Rescue Remedy cream to sore nipples, but wipe before feeding.

✳ For **insufficient lactation**, drink fennel tea or eat fennel seeds. This may also relieve colic in the baby.

See page 150–1 for further information

POSTNATAL

Care of the Perineum

DURING DELIVERY, THE PERINEUM STRETCHES to its fullest extent. It may tear if the baby is large, the perineum is tight, or delivery is rapid. Occasionally, an episiotomy is necessary. This is a surgical incision that is stitched after the birth. There are many natural treatments to aid healing: combine them with good nutrition and personal hygiene.

POSSIBLE PROBLEMS

Pain and soreness from tears or stitches

✳

Bruising and inflammation

✳

Infection of tear or stitches and slow healing

REFLEXOLOGY

Foot massage can stimulate the body's natural healing powers and promote a feeling of well-being during the recovery period after the birth of your baby. If you are in a great deal of discomfort as a result of a perineal tear or an episiotomy, it might be more appropriate to have treatment administered by a practitioner than to use self-help measures.

✳ The reflex points corresponding to the perineum, the pelvic area or the lymphatic system may be appropriate for treatment of the perineum.

See page 140–1 for further information

KEY TIPS

Eat healthily to promote healing

✳

Clean and dry the area after using the toilet

✳

Change pads frequently

FOOT MASSAGE
A reflexology treatment is preceded by a massage that relaxes the foot and reveals areas of tenderness corresponding to health problems.

CAUTIONS

If a stitch is pulling, your midwife might be able to remove it to make you more comfortable. If you develop fever, chills, extreme fatigue, flu-like symptoms or the perineum does not seem to be healing, consult your doctor.

POSTNATAL

COMPLEMENTARY TREATMENTS

Before using a complementary treatment, please read any **Cautions** and the relevant page references

PARTICULARLY IF YOUR PERINEUM HAS BEEN STITCHED, help to prevent infection by eating healthily in order to boost the immune system. High standards of personal hygiene are essential. A sore perineum can be treated with ultrasound or pulsed electromagnetic energy (megapulse), which relieves pain and reduces swelling. Hold a polythene bag filled with crushed ice to the area to reduce swelling but only for ten minutes as it might restrict circulation. When breastfeeding, sit on a pillow or lie on your side. When resting or in bed, lie on your back with a pillow under your bottom to relieve pressure on the perineum, or lie on your side with a pillow between your knees. Start doing pelvic floor exercises as soon as you can to improve local circulation and thus promote healing.

ACUPUNCTURE

This treatment can be of benefit in relieving **pain and soreness** in the perineum.

✳ Ear acupuncture can be beneficial for perineal **tears and stitches**. The acupoint that relates to the external genitalia is stimulated.

✳ A TENS machine (*see page 109*) may help to ease perineal discomfort. The pads should be placed on the acupoints GV1 to either side of the coccyx.

See pages 134–5 for further information

HOMEOPATHY

Continue to take *Arnica 6c*, as you did before the birth (as directed) as a preventative measure or to reduce **bruising and inflammation** of the perineum.

See pages 148–9 for further information

FLOWER REMEDIES

Gentle flower remedies may help to ease you through the emotional turmoil of the postnatal period.

✳ Crab apple is recommended if the soreness of your perineum and the general state of your postnatal body is making you feel unpleasant and "unclean".

See page 154 for further information

CRAB APPLE
The remedy made from this flower brings relief to those women who feel despondent after the birth.

AROMATHERAPY

A few drops of lavender, calendula or tea tree oils added to your bath will help to soothe the **soreness** after stitches or a tear.

See pages 152–3 for further information

WESTERN HERBALISM

There are a number of herbal remedies to promote the healing of the perineum.

✳ Apply soothing calendula lotion, even on broken skin.

✳ Add an appropriate tincture to a bath or bidet: chamomile for **bruising and inflammation**; marigold to alleviate soreness; and arnica to reduce bruising and **soreness** and promote healing. Add salt to prevent **infection** and promote healing.

See pages 150–1 for further information

NUTRITION

It is essential after the blood loss during birth to replace vital nutrients. Eat foods rich in:

✳ Vitamin C, for skin repair and iron absorption. Good food sources include citrus fruits and broccoli.

✳ Zinc, for hormone production and healing. Good food sources include fish, poultry and wholegrains.

See pages 116–17 for further information

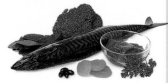

IRON-RICH FOODS
Eating such foods will promote healing and fight infection.

POSTNATAL

Caesarean Section

How you feel emotionally and physically after a Caesarean section will depend largely on whether you had an elective (planned) or an emergency section (rushed into theatre because of concerns about you or the baby). The latter can leave you feeling shocked and emotional and you are more likely to have had a general anaesthetic.

AROMATHERAPY

An aromatherapy treatment may help to relieve headaches, nausea and vomiting, the possible side effects of anaesthetic. **Infection** can sometimes occur in the wound following a Caesarean section. If it is inflamed and you have a temperature and flu-like symptoms, you will need antibiotics, but a few drops of eucalyptus oil in a foot bath may help to relieve your general discomfort.

✱ If you have a **headache**, rub a couple of drops of essential oil of lavender (undiluted) into each temple.
✱ For relief from **nausea and vomiting**, sniff essential oil of peppermint.

See page 152–3 for further information

SOOTHING A HEADACHE
Sit in a comfortable position, close your eyes and try to relax completely before gently rubbing lavender oil into your temples.

KEY TIPS

Get as much rest and sleep as possible to aid healing and general recuperation
✱
Allow yourself time to recover properly and do not attempt to do too much
✱
Eat a healthy diet that includes zinc-rich foods since this mineral is rapidly used up in the healing process

CAUTION

If you develop fever, chills, extreme fatigue, flu-like symptoms or your wound is inflamed and does not seem to be healing properly you may have an infection and should consult your doctor.

POSTNATAL

COMPLEMENTARY TREATMENTS

Before using a complementary treatment, please read any **Cautions** and relevant page references

COMPLEMENTARY TREATMENTS may help to ease a variety of discomforts following a Caesarean section. If you had a general anaesthetic, you may feel quite "out of it" on day one. You will have an intravenous infusion running and a urinary catheter bag. You may be given intramuscular injections for pain relief. The best thing to do is rest, sleep and cuddle your baby. A physiotherapist may help you to start gentle circulatory exercises in bed and deep breathing exercises will enable you to clear congestion following a general anaesthetic. The next day you may be able to get up and take a shower. The catheter will be removed to see if you can pass urine naturally. You will by now be taking pain relief orally, as required. Make sure you are comfortable for breastfeeding. You may feel emotional on day three, especially following an emergency section. Rest and sleep as much as possible on day four, even if you feel better, since you may be allowed home the following day.

HOMEOPATHY

Homeopathic remedies may help to ease both physical and emotional problems after a Caesarean section:

✻ Many women feel tearful after surgery, especially a Caesarean. Take *Arnica 6c* to help to stabilize your emotions and *Aconite 6c* for shock.

✻ If you feel drowsy and spaced-out after the anaesthetic, take *Opium 6c*.

See pages 148–9 for further information

EASY TO TAKE
Remedies in pill form are taken from the container.

WESTERN HERBALISM

Many women who have had a Caesarean section, especially an elective one, experience **insufficient lactation**. Their milk may take longer to come in because the hormones triggered by spontaneous labour are not activated in the same way.

✻ Drink fennel tea to encourage milk production.

See pages 150–1 for further information

FLOWER REMEDIES

Flower remedies may bring gentle relief at an emotionally demanding time.

✻ If you feel **tearful** and highly emotional, Rescue Remedy or Five Flower Remedy may help to calm you.

✻ If you are suffering from **exhaustion**, try olive.

See page 154 for further information

TENS MACHINE

If your wound is very sore, a TENS machine can provide effective natural pain relief. Place two pads above the scar and two below the scar. These can be left in place indefinitely.

See page 109 for further information

NUTRITION

A good diet is important following a Caesarean section. Take a daily multivitamin and eat plenty of foods rich in vitamin C, iron and zinc to encourage your body to fight infection, to help your wound to heal, and to prevent anaemia (if you have lost a lot of blood). In addition:

✻ Take energy-rich drinks and light meals or snacks regularly.

✻ Take a DHA supplement if you are breastfeeding.

See pages 116–17 for further information

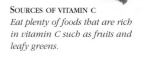

SOURCES OF VITAMIN C
Eat plenty of foods that are rich in vitamin C such as fruits and leafy greens.

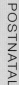

POSTNATAL

POSTNATAL DEPRESSION

WOMEN SUFFER FROM POSTNATAL DEPRESSION for a variety of biological, psychological and social reasons. Exhaustion is often the main cause of depression immediately following delivery and for the next few weeks. However, the difficult period sometimes comes at about four months, when much support that was originally there is no longer available.

REIKI

Reiki is a wonderfully healing and balancing treatment for body, mind and spirit. Postnatally it can help to bring you back into yourself, releasing traumatic feelings resulting from the birth. A reiki practitioner will treat you and, if you like, teach you how to treat yourself.

See page 139 for further information

See page 139 for further information

KEY TIPS

Do not try to over-achieve: set yourself realistic targets
✳
Accept offers of help
✳
Find 10–20 minutes for yourself each day
✳
Eat a balanced diet
✳
Do not deny your feelings: seek help if you need it

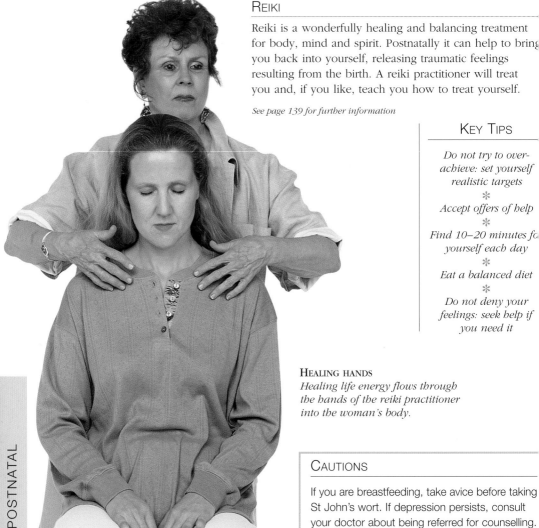

HEALING HANDS
Healing life energy flows through the hands of the reiki practitioner into the woman's body.

CAUTIONS

If you are breastfeeding, take avice before taking St John's wort. If depression persists, consult your doctor about being referred for counselling.

POSTNATAL

COMPLEMENTARY TREATMENTS

Before using a complementary treatment, please read any **Cautions** and the relevant page references

COMPLEMENTARY TREATMENTS can help postnatal depression, but you should also consider diet. The condition is exacerbated or even partially caused by hormone imbalances and chemical changes, the effects of which can be reduced by good nutrition. Copper levels rise naturally during pregnancy and peak after delivery. This is offset if zinc levels are high, but these may have been seriously depleted. Excessive copper and zinc deficiency are believed to contribute to postnatal depression. Take a zinc supplement, plus vitamins B^6 and C.

ACUPUNCTURE

If you had a traumatic delivery, acupuncture can help to "settle your spirit". Treatment is based on nourishing the Blood, improving the flow of *qi* and calming the mind. Certain acupoints may be used to release neurotransmitters that help relieve depression.

See pages 134–5 for further information

WESTERN HERBALISM

Certain plants have a reputation for being able to lift the spirits.

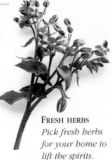

✳ Drink teas such as lemon balm, peppermint or orange blossom for a "lift".

✳ Take St John's wort to alleviate depression.

See pages 150–1 for further information

FRESH HERBS
Pick fresh herbs for your home to lift the spirits.

AROMATHERAPY

A massage using lavender or citrus oils may relax you and encourage a feeling of well-being, thus reducing depression.

✳ Burn essential oils of jasmine, lemon, lime or grapefruit in a room to invigorate you.

✳ Have a long soak in a warm bath to which a few drops of any of the above-mentioned oils have been added.

Caution: see page 153 for oils to avoid.

See pages 152–3 for further information

SHIATSU & REFLEXOLOGY

Both treatments use the stimulation of pressure points to help to relieve postnatal depression. The postnatal period is believed by the Chinese to be a "gateway of change", a crucial time when a woman must take care of herself and replenish her energy.

See pages 138 and 140–1 for further information

FLOWER REMEDIES

Many flower remedies are suitable for the relief of a variety of feelings that you might experience after the birth of your baby. Those most appropriate for despondency and depression include the following.

✳ Mustard, for inexplicable depression.

✳ Gentian, if you know why you are depressed and you feel despondent and discouraged.

✳ Sweet chestnut, if you are desperate.

✳ Clematis, if you feel detached from reality.

✳ Red chestnut, if you are over-anxious.

✳ Pine, if you need to regain perspective and if you feel guilty as if you have failed in some way.

✳ Elm, if you feel overwhelmed by the responsibilities of parenthood.

✳ Crab apple, to ease trauma and feelings of self-loathing and self-disgust.

See page 154 for further information

PSYCHOTHERAPY & COUNSELLING

Cognitive behavioural therapy can help you to turn pessimistic thoughts into positive ones and relieve mild or moderate depression. Counselling will help you to work through feelings arising from your depression.

POSTNATAL

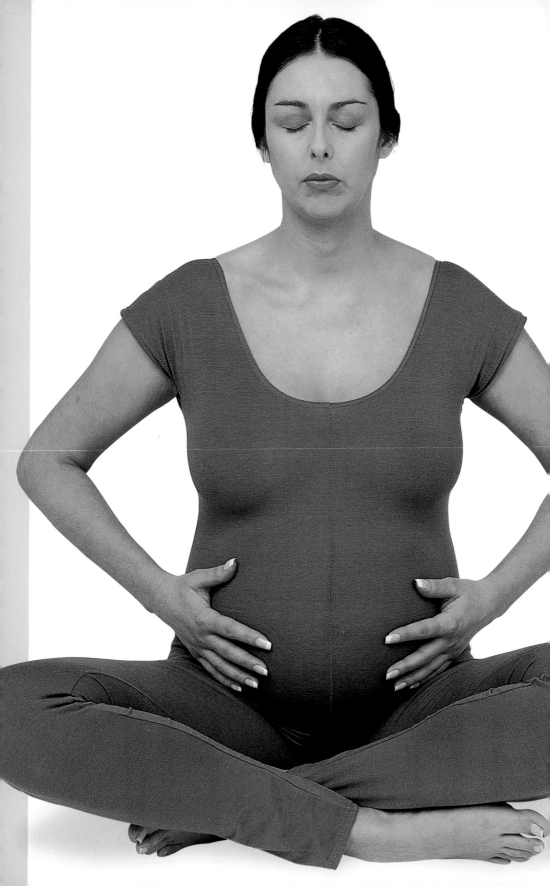

THERE IS A WEALTH of complementary therapies and natural treatments available for the relief of minor ailments during pregnancy and to maximize your body's constitutional strength, thus enabling you to enjoy your pregnancy in as healthy a physical and mental state as possible. If you are unfamiliar with complementary

Complementary therapies

therapies, and reluctant to try them out in pregnancy, this chapter aims to give you a basic understanding of the treatments recommended in the preceding sections. It seeks to remove any concerns that you might have about safety and suitability so that you can confidently choose the therapy that is right for you.

Traditional Chinese Beliefs

ACCORDING TO TRADITIONAL CHINESE MEDICINE (TCM), *qi*, or "vital energy", is the key life force. It flows around the body in meridians, or channels, and is the catalyst for every metabolic change, movement, sensation and thought. Good health is the result of living in accordance with the flow of energy in the body.

USES IN PREGNANCY

✻ *General guidance on healthy living and mental well-being*

THE 24-HOUR BODY CLOCK

Practitioners of Traditional Chinese Medicine look for a pattern of symptoms, rather a specific disease. If an organ in the body is deficient in *qi*, symptoms of an ailment appear during that organ's low-energy, or "rest", period. Each period in a 24-hour cycle relates to an organ (*see below*). The following are the peak periods for each.

• 7 am to 9 am Stomach. The Chinese believe that you should "eat like a prince at breakfast, a merchant at lunch and a pauper at dinner".

• 9 am to 11 am Spleen and the transportation of food and ideas. A short walk helps *qi* to flow and aids the digestive process. This is the most productive part of your day.

• 11 am to 1 pm Heart. This is the best time of day to engage in aerobic exercise.

• 1 pm to 3 pm Small Intestine, which is associated with mental activity. This is when you will be at your sharpest mentally.

• 3 pm to 5 pm Bladder. This is the time to draw your day's activities to a close.

• 5 pm to 7 pm Kidneys, which are associated with reproduction. If your pregnancy is considered high risk, or if you have oedema or high blood pressure, rest at this time.

• 7 pm to 9 pm Pericardium, which is associated with opennesss and relating to people. This is a good time to meet with friends and family.

• 9 pm to 11 pm is the peak time for the "Triple Burner" – an organ with no physical form but which harmonizes the upper, middle and lower body and influences body fluids and

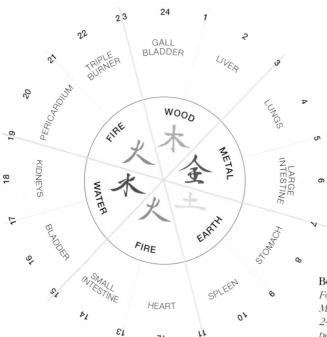

BODY CYCLES
Followers of Traditional Chinese Medicine believe that during each 24-hour cycle, every organ in the body peaks for a two-hour period, then has a period of low energy 12 hours later.

火

One element either supports or inhibits another: so water douses fire, while fire melts metal. Similarly, one organ affects another: the Kidneys control the Heart, while the Heart controls the Lungs.

木

FIRE
Season: summer
Taste: bitter
Emotion: joy
Parts of the body: Heart, Small intestine, Tongue, Blood vessels

土

WOOD
Season: spring
Taste: sour
Emotion: anger
Parts of the body: Liver, Gall bladder, Tendons, Eyes

EARTH
Season: late summer
Taste: sweet
Emotion: worry
Parts of the body: Spleen, Stomach, Mouth, Muscles

the flow of *qi*. Everything slows now ready for sleep.
• 11 pm to 1 am Gall Bladder. This is the time in which to sleep and dream.
• 1 am to 3 am Liver and detoxification.
• 3 am to 5 am Lungs. This is the peak time for dreaming.
• 5 am to 7 am Large Intestine. This is the best time of day to open the bowels.

水

金

WATER
Season: winter
Taste: salty
Emotion: fear
Parts of the body: Kidneys, Bladder, Ears, Bones

METAL
Season: autumn
Taste: pungent
Emotion: grief
Parts of the body: Lungs, Large intestine, Nose, Skin

SEASONAL HARMONY

The concept of living in harmony with nature is an ancient one and fundamental to TCM. The seasons of the year and the changes they bring about affect our growth and well-being. Think of your pregnancy as lasting for 12 months, including three months of preconceptual care. To keep good health, you need to live in harmony with the seasons and adjust your diet, exercise and lifestyle habits accordingly. Spring and summer are *yang* months – a time of warmth, growth and activity, while autumn and winter are *ying* months – a time for harvesting and storage, rest and reflection.

FIVE-ELEMENT THEORY

Traditional Chinese beliefs also hold that the five elements fire, earth, metal, wood and water are symbolic of all things in the

universe. These elements are used by practitioners as touchstones in prescribing for specific ailments. Disorders in organs linked with a specific element are treated with herbs corresponding to that element. Each element is associated with a particular season, certain physical activities (*see page 19*), a *yin* and a *yang* organ, a taste and an emotion.
• Spring is associated with the Liver and Gall Bladder and the element wood. It is strongly linked to birth and growth. This is a good time of year for cleansing, starting afresh with new plans, and mental exercise. Consume plenty of water, green vegetables, juices and seeds.
• Summer is associated with the Heart, Small Intestine, Pericardium and Triple Burner

and the element fire. This is the time for outdoor activity and for eating fruit and salad vegetables.
• Late summer is associated with the Stomach and Spleen and the element earth. This is a time for grounding, centring, meditating and building up strength. Eat plenty of fruit, berries, nuts and seeds.
• Autumn is associated with the Lungs and Large Intestine and the element metal. Now is the time to wind down and turn inwards in preparation for winter. Eat berries such as blackcurrants and blackberries.
• Winter is associated with the Kidneys and Bladder and the element water. This is the time for hibernation and inward reflection, keeping warm and building up energy. Eat root vegetables and cooked grains.

Acupuncture

ACUPUNCTURE IS PART OF TRADITIONAL CHINESE MEDICINE, dating back 3,500 years. Practitioners believe that vital energy (*qi*) flows through the body along invisible channels called meridians. If *qi* circulates freely, you are in good health: if circulation is disrupted, illness results. Acupuncture can regulate the flow of *qi*.

USES IN PREGNANCY

* *Morning sickness*
* *Threatened miscarriage*
* *Heartburn*
* *Migraine*
* *Varicose veins*
* *Postnatal depression*

HOW IT WORKS

According to Traditional Chinese Medicine (*see pages 132–3*), *qi* is created in the body by the interaction of the opposite but complementary forces of *yin* and *yang*. For the body to be healthy, *yin* and *yang* must be in balance (*tao*). *Yin* signifies cold, damp, and contraction, while *yang* signifies heat, dryness and inflammation. Illness arises if *yin* and *yang* are not in equilibrium so that the flow of *qi* is disrupted. Ancient Chinese healers discovered that the stimulation of distinct points on the body both allays pain and affects the functioning of their corresponding organs. These 365 points, called acupoints, are not scattered randomly but follow an unchanging pattern. The line linking the acupoints that are associated with a particular organ – the Spleen, Liver, Lungs and so on – is known as a meridian. To treat the symptoms of ailments and relieve pain, fine needles are inserted at specific acupoints along the relevant meridians. Chinese healers claim that acupuncture works either by encouraging or suppressing the flow of *qi* along these meridians. Western scientists believe that acupuncture works by altering the body's normal pain response in some way.

DIAGNOSIS

Your first appointment with an acupuncturist may take up to 90 minutes. The practitioner will take a detailed medical history. Everything about you is relevant: lifestyle, emotions and physical characteristics,

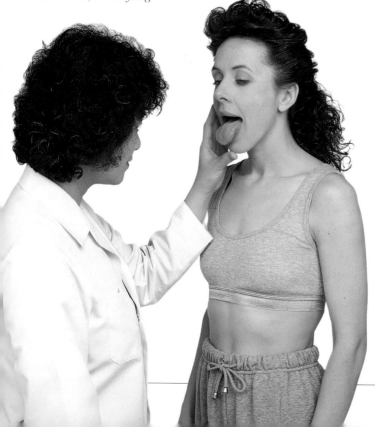

TONGUE DIAGNOSIS
The colour and coatings of the tongue are said to reflect your state of health as a whole.

as well as the symptoms of the condition needing treatment. All the body's systems are considered, especially digestion and circulation, as well as sleep patterns and energy levels. Some aspects of diagnosis may seem unusual. Your tongue will be carefully examined, for example, since different areas are believed to relate to different organs, and various coatings and colours are indicative of particular ailments.

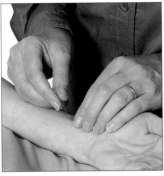

TAKING YOUR PULSES
An acupuncturist reads three pulse points on each wrist of the patient. Traditional Chinese Medicine holds that there are 28 possible types of pulse.

A yellow coating, for instance, is said to indicate excessive internal "heat", which would need to be cleared, while a white coating indicates excessive "cold". Pulse-taking is another important diagnostic tool of the acupuncturist. The flow of *qi* and the balance of *yin* and *yang* are said to be reflected in three pulse points along the radial artery at each wrist. All the pulse points are checked and compared for strength and rhythm using the application of light, moderate and heavy

pressure. The relative differences between them indicate the degree of equilibrium in the flow of *qi*.

TREATMENT

An acupuncturist treats a patient holistically, and each treatment will be tailored to your individual needs. Usually, four or six needles are left in place for between 15 and 20 minutes, but sometimes for longer. You may experience a slight tingling sensation or even a dull ache. A feeling of relaxation usually follows, but be aware that symptoms may appear to intensify before they start to improve.

OTHER TECHNIQUES

Another technique used in Traditional Chinese Medicine to encourage a balanced flow of *qi* is moxabustion. This uses the herb moxa, the Chinese name for mugwort (*Artemesia vulgaris*), which is dried and rolled into a stick or cone. A stick is lit, like a cigar, and held over an acupoint in order to stimulate it until the skin becomes uncomfortably hot. Moxa cones are lit, placed directly on acupoints and left to smoulder on the skin, again until the heat is uncomfortable. Moxa can also be put in a steel burner attached to a needle head. These methods of transferring heat to acupoints are generally used to remedy conditions that are associated with a deficiency in *qi* or with "cold". Moxibustion can be used in pregnancy, and is even believed to be able to help to re-orientate a breech baby that is poorly positioned for birth.

TAKING CARE

If you are considering having acupuncture treatment before you become pregnant, you must inform your practitioner that you are trying to conceive. As with all complementary therapies in pregnancy, make sure that the acupuncturist you consult is fully qualified. Certain acupoints should not be stimulated in pregnancy, except during labour. Avoid contact with heavy metals, drinking alcohol, eating a large meal, having a hot bath or shower or taking strenuous exercise (including sex) before or after an acupuncture treatment to avoid counteracting its effects.

AURICULAR ACUPUNCTURE

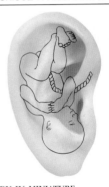

BODY IN MINIATURE
In TCM the ear is highly significant. Said to resemble an inverted foetus, it has more than 120 acupoints and is crossed by all major meridians. During auricular (ear) acupuncture, the ear is examined very carefully, especially the condition and colour of the skin. Gentle pressure is applied to the relevant acupoint with the fingers or tiny acupuncture needles. Modern techniques include the use of lasers.

Acupressure

ACUPRESSURE IS ACUPUNTURE without needles. As part of Traditional Chinese Medicine, it is based on the same principles as acupuncture. It is highly appropriate for people who are afraid of needles and has great self-help potential for the treatment of some of the common ailments of pregnancy.

USES IN PREGNANCY

* *Morning sickness*
* *Backache & Sciatica*
* *Stress & Anxiety*
* *Fatigue*

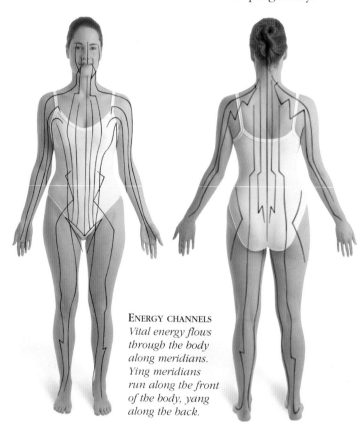

ENERGY CHANNELS
Vital energy flows through the body along meridians. Ying meridians run along the front of the body, yang along the back.

and sciatica, migraine, heartburn, constipation and carpal tunnel syndrome, for induction and during labour.

TREATMENT & SELF-HELP

A practitioner will study your medical history and assess your symptoms. He or she will then apply pressure to the relevant point, angling the fingers and thumbs in the direction of the meridian for maximum effect. You can learn how to use the technique yourself to relieve ailments. Certain applications, such as using the Pericardium meridian to treat morning sickness (*see page 37*), have been successful, but in general acupressure is considered less effective than acupuncture. It can be effective, however, as a self-help back-up measure between acupuncture sessions.

TAKING CARE

Make sure that you consult a fully qualified practitioner. As with acupuncture, there are guidelines that warn against the application of pressure to certain acupoints at particular stages of pregnancy, and these need to be explained to you.

HOW IT WORKS

Acupressure is regularly used in China to treat common ailments. Based on the belief that *qi* flows around the body along meridians (*see page 134*), finger pressure is applied to the relevant acupoints to relieve symptoms and establish balance within the body. The Japanese system of healing, shiatsu, is founded on the same principles. During pregnancy, acupressure may be useful for the treatment of morning sickness, hyperemesis, backache

T'ai Chi

T'AI CHI IS A NON-COMBATIVE MARTIAL ART that uses a series of movements combined with breathing techniques to improve the flow of *qi* in the body, calm the mind and encourage the body's own powers of self-healing. It is practised daily by people of all ages in China and is increasingly popular in the West.

> ### USES IN PREGNANCY
>
> * *Stress & Anxiety*
> * *Fatigue*
> * *Exercise*
> * *Relaxation*

HOW IT WORKS

T'ai chi ch'uan, which is usually known simply as t'ai chi, is a movement therapy intended to ensure an uninterrupted flow of *qi*, or "vital energy", around the body through meridians (*see page 134*). There are five styles of t'ai chi. In the most popular version, *Yang*, the participant executes a series of postures that are evocative of animals, martial stances and natural forms. Each posture flows into the next, creating a rhythmic and powerful sequence that is designed to focus mind and body in harmony in order to improve the flow of *qi*. The "short form" of the discipline involves 24 movements and takes about ten minutes, while the "long form" can take up to 40 minutes. T'ai chi is ideally practised outdoors so that the earth's *qi* can link with that of the body.

T'AI CHI & PREGNANCY

This therapy is designed to relax muscles and nerves – thus ultimately benefitting all body systems – and improve posture, balance and the flexibility of joints. It therefore has great potential for use during pregnancy. While it may be safely practised in all three trimesters, it is best to begin developing balance and strengthening muscles and joints in the early stages. You can teach yourself t'ai chi from a video, but it is advisable during pregnancy to take instruction from a qualified teacher, who will also be able to explain the philosophy behind the therapy and point out postures that should be avoided as you approach full term. T'ai chi provides a gentle form of exercise that many pregnant women will find suitable for them. Its relaxation and breathing techniques are useful for the relief of stress-related ailments as well as for the improvement of mental and physical control, which may be particularly valuable in pregnancy and labour.

TAKING CARE

Make sure that your teacher is aware of your pregnancy and any medical conditions before you start a class. Always begin your exercise routine with a gentle warm-up and do not over-exert yourself.

LEARNING TECHNIQUE
A qualified instructor will ensure that your t'ai chi stance is correct in order to maximise the benefits of the therapy and maintain postures that are suitable for pregnancy.

Shiatsu

SHIATSU TRANSLATES LITERALLY from the Japanese as "finger pressure". A system of healing through touch, with roots in Traditional Chinese Medicine, the technique evolved in Japan in the 19th century from a synthesis of traditional massage techniques and Western knowledge of physiology.

USES IN PREGNANCY

＊ *Morning sickness*
＊ *Backache & Sciatica*
＊ *Sleeplessness*
＊ *Raised blood pressure*
＊ *Oedema*

HOW IT WORKS

At its highest level, shiatsu combines finely-tuned intuition with a thorough understanding of the structure of the body. Like acupuncture (*see pages 134–5*), its principles are based on improving the flow of vital energy (*ki* in Japanese) through the internal organs of the body and their meridians. Vitality is seen as the basis of health, and it reflects the strength and

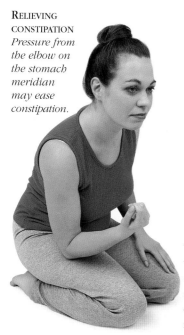

RELIEVING CONSTIPATION
Pressure from the elbow on the stomach meridian may ease constipation.

harmony of *ki* circulation. Practitioners attempt to boost and correct disturbances in the flow of *ki* by means of a series of manipulations, with the intention of either unblocking constricted energy flow or stemming excess flow, as is required. These measures are believed to regulate nerve function, strengthen resistence to disease, "flush out" the organ or tissue in question, improve blood circulation and make joints more flexible.

DIAGNOSIS & TREATMENT

A shiatsu consultation lasts up to an hour. At your first visit, the practitioner will take a detailed medical history as well as examining your tongue, observing your posture and taking your pulse. The *hara* diagnosis technique is one of the most important parts of the consultation. Centred on the abdominal area, *hara* "maps" the energy in the body. The practitioner will palpate your abdomen gently to determine the energetic state and condition of internal organs and their corresponding meridians. A shiatsu treatment

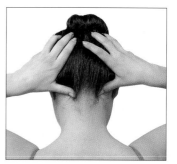

EASING A HEADACHE
Applying pressure to Gallbladder 20 acupoint is a useful self-help measure to relieve a headache.

involves the therapist gently stretching, holding and leaning his or her body weight into various parts of your body. Pressure is applied through the hands, thumbs, fingers, forearms, knees and feet as you sit or lie in various positions.

TAKING CARE

Choose a practitioner who has experience of treating pregnant women and who is aware of acupoints that should not be used during massage in pregnancy. Avoid drinking alcohol, eating a large meal, having a hot bath or shower or strenuous exercise just before or after a shiatsu treatment.

Reiki

LOOSELY TRANSLATED, reiki means "universal life energy". This method of spiritual healing is based on ancient Tibetan Buddhist teachings, and was formulated after years of research, travel and meditation by Dr Mikao Usui, a Japanese theologian. It is claimed to promote health and well-being but is clinically unproven.

USES IN PREGNANCY

* ✱ *Backache & Sciatica*
* ✱ *Headaches*
* ✱ *Stress & Anxiety*
* ✱ *Postnatal depression*

HOW IT WORKS

A simple technique, yet one that is claimed to be very powerful, reiki is practised by masters whose lives are committed to this work and the lifestyle that it engenders. When activated and applied for the purpose of healing, reiki energy flows through their hands to wherever it is needed in the patient's body. The therapy addresses physical, mental and spiritual well-being, accelerating the body's own powers of healing and balance. According to reiki masters, the body responds to treatment in the same way that a plant takes up water – absorbing it if needed, or not at all. Healing energy travels straight to the source of any problem, dislodging harmful "blockages" and rebalancing energy flow. This generates a feeling of profound release, which in turn promotes deep relaxation, mental and emotional harmony and relief from ailments. It is believed that deeper causes of problems will become apparent as reiki is performed, thus paving the way for change. After treatment, both patient and practitioner feel revitalized.

TREATMENT

A reiki treatment takes about an hour. The practitioner will hold his or her hands on or above your body in 12 positions. In pregnancy, it may be helpful in easing back pain and morning sickness. If given regularly, it is also said to encourage smooth labour. In the postnatal period, the treatment is effective on a spiritual and emotional level, bringing the mother "home" into herself, calming distressed babies and easing birth trauma.

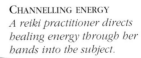

CHANNELLING ENERGY
A reiki practitioner directs healing energy through her hands into the subject.

Reflexology

RELATED TO ANCIENT TECHNIQUES of foot massage, this therapy is based on the theory that reflex points on the feet act as nerve receptors for all organs of the body, to which they are linked by energy pathways. Reflexology works well in conjunction with orthodox treatment for common ailments in pregnancy.

USES IN PREGNANCY

* *Morning sickness*
* *Backache*
* *Migraine*
* *Constipation*
* *Cystitis*
* *Raised blood pressure*

HOW IT WORKS

The system of reflexology used today evolved from the work of Dr William Fitzgerald, an American ear, nose and throat specialist. In 1915, he discovered that applying pressure to certain areas of the body produced a numbing effect in areas far removed from the pressure point. He hypothesized that energy moves from the extremities toward the head in distinct channels or zones, and that any disorder within a given zone can be treated by working on a corresponding area on the foot or the hand. Today, reflexologists focus primarily on the feet. They believe that pressure applied to specific reflex points highlights past, current or potential energy disturbances, and that treatment in the form of massage helps to smooth out these disturbances or blockages and stimulate the body's self-healing capacity.

Although reflexology is not a diagnostic tool, it is possible to detect disorders or diseased areas. It does not aim to treat illness specifically, but to stimulate the body's innate capacity to rebalance and heal itself. Both physical and emotional problems are said to respond to reflexology. While medical doctors are largely sceptical about the therapy's ability to remedy physical conditions, reflexology is demonstrably effective for relaxation and the relief of stress, allowing the body to re-establish its equilibrium.

DIAGNOSIS

A reflexologist will first take a detailed medical history. Before treatment, you will be asked to remove your shoes and socks. When examining your feet, a

SELF-HELP REFLEXOLOGY
Stimulating the solar plexus reflex point below the ball of the foot may help stem nausea.

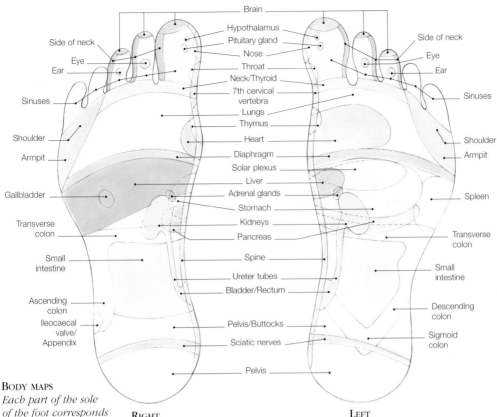

Brain
Hypothalamus
Pituitary gland
Nose
Side of neck
Eye
Ear
Throat
Neck/Thyroid
7th cervical
vertebra
Sinuses
Lungs
Thymus
Shoulder
Heart
Armpit
Diaphragm
Solar plexus
Liver
Gallbladder
Adrenal glands
Stomach
Kidneys
Transverse
colon
Pancreas
Small
intestine
Spine
Ureter tubes
Bladder/Rectum
Ascending
colon
Ileocaecal
valve/
Appendix
Pelvis/Buttocks
Sciatic nerves
Pelvis

Side of neck
Eye
Ear
Sinuses
Shoulder
Armpit
Spleen
Transverse
colon
Small
intestine
Descending
colon
Sigmoid
colon

RIGHT   **LEFT**

BODY MAPS
*Each part of the sole
of the foot corresponds
to a different part of the
body. A reflexologist
reads the foot rather like a
map, identifying regions of
tenderness as manifestations of
ailments elsewhere in the body.*

practitioner will seek evidence
of ill-health, for example
discolouration, swelling,
dry patches or rashes. Your
sensitivity to touch is also
considered to be significant.
Therapists believe that waste
products accumulate around
vulnerable reflex points,
causing tenderness, which
indicates blocked energy
flow elsewhere in the body.

TREATMENT

During a treatment, a therapist's
thumbs or fingers move across
the toes and soles, covering
every reflex point. By pinching,
stroking and clasping, attempts
are made to disperse "toxic
deposits" and thus free up
energy flow. You may feel a
bruised or pricking sensation
when work is being done on
areas of the foot relating to
affected organs. Each treatment
can take up to an hour or more,
and six weekly sessions are
usually recommended as a
course of treatment. Some
reflexology techniques can be
taught as self-help measures.
A therapist may instruct you
so that you can treat yourself
at home. Despite little scientific
verification, it has been claimed
anecdotally that more than 100
different ailments can benefit
from reflexology.

TAKING PRECAUTIONS

As with most therapies, if you
have any history of miscarriage
or if there is a risk of foetal loss
or major placental disturbance,
such as placenta previa or pre-
eclampsia, you should avoid
reflexology. Great care should
be taken in the first three
months of pregnancy and with
a first treatment at any time
during pregnancy. Tell the
practitioner if you are taking
any medication. If you are
in any doubt about using
reflexology while you are
pregnant, consult your midwife
or doctor. If you are using
self-help techniques and are
concerned about any aspect
of your condition, consult a
qualified reflexologist.

Yoga

YOGA IS A SANSKRIT WORD, meaning union. The discipline originated in India more than 5,000 years ago and was propounded by Hindu ascetics. Brought to the West in the 19th century, it has found a widespread following. Yoga can be very useful in pregnancy, labour and the postnatal period.

USES IN PREGNANCY

* *Morning sickness*
* *Backache*
* *Haemorrhoids/Varicose veins*
* *Depression*
* *Breech baby*
* *Respiratory problems*

HOW IT WORKS

Many people think of yoga merely as a gentle form of breathing exercise, but it is in fact a complex system of physical and mental training. Highly beneficial during pregnancy and postnatally, it is the preferred form of exercise of increasing numbers of expectant women and new mothers. Yoga is used for strengthening, toning and relaxing; to open up the pelvis before the birth and recover good muscle tone after it. There are many different systems of yoga, but they all confer physical and spiritual benefits. More esoteric forms of yoga concentrate on the body's centres of life energy, or *chakras*. Focusing on the *chakras* during yoga and meditation influences the flow of life energy, or *prana*, through the "subtle", or non-physical, body. One of the most popular forms of yoga in the West is *hatha*, which uses *asanas*, or postures, and *pranayamas*, or breathing techniques, to encourage calm, relaxation and balance between body and mind.

FINDING A TEACHER

There are many yoga classes available, some of which are specifically designed for pregnant women. The teachers of these will be aware of the physiological changes that occur during pregnancy and can suggest positions that are comfortable and appropriate for pregnant women. One-to-one tuition is also available. Yoga has great self-help potential once you are familiar with the postures and breathing methods.

TAKING CARE

Listen to your body and avoid positions that do not feel comfortable. Stop if you are in pain or if you feel unwell. Do gentle movements up to 14 weeks and do not exercise flat on your back after 30 weeks. Some yoga teachers do not recommend its use during the first trimester of pregnancy.

BODY & MIND
Sitting in a relaxed, cross-legged position and breathing deeply promotes calm, which has important physical benefits.

Meditation & Visualization

MEDITATION IS A MEANS of inducing profound relaxation and heightened awareness, thus counteracting stress-related conditions. Visualization, too, is a technique that enables people to cope with stressful situations and encourages the body's self-healing mechanisms. Both these practices can be of help during pregnancy.

USES IN PREGNANCY

* *Morning sickness*
* *Threatened miscarriage*
* *Sleeplessness*
* *Stress & Anxiety*
* *Raised blood pressure*
* *During labour*

MEDITATION

The meditative technique of emptying the mind while focusing on a thought or image encourages a health-enhancing "relaxation response" in the body. One of the most popular techniques is Transcendental Meditation, based on Hindu philosophy. During meditation alpha brainwaves are produced. These are associated with deep relaxation, lowered blood pressure, decreased muscle tension and less stress.

VISUALIZATION

This technique can also be used to relieve stress. In early pregnancy many women find it difficult to connect with their baby, especially if they feel unwell with morning sickness. This may cause resentment and anxiety. Relating to your baby does not happen automatically; it has to be worked at. It is worth taking time each day to sit with your hands on your stomach, visualizing the unborn child and thinking positive thoughts about your future together. Visualization can also be used to cope with painful contractions during labour.

LEARNING TECHNIQUES

You can learn most meditative and visualization techniques from books or videos, or you can consult a practitioner, either on a one-to-one basis or in a group. You may feel that tuition is more appropriate, but

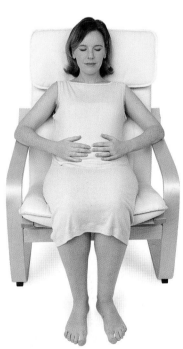

SITTING COMFORTABLY
Sit in a chair that supports the whole body so that you can relax fully and concentrate the mind.

techniques are generally easy to follow at home. These therapies require a quiet place where you can sit or lie and relax. Relaxation is fundamental. Breathe slowly, steadily and rhythmically, inhaling through the nose and exhaling through the mouth. Repeat a mantra or focus totally on an object of meditation such as a flower or a candle. If you are using visualization as means of stress relief, imagine a pleasing scene such as a tropical beach or a mountain vista, or imagine the birth going really well.

TAKING CARE

Check with your doctor before starting to practice meditation or visualization if you have any history of psychiatric illness or a medical condition that may be exacerbated by the emergence of images of a potentially disturbing nature. Consult a qualified practitioner in these disciplines if you are at all concerned about the techniques involved and how they might affect your baby or if you notice a deterioration in any of your symptoms if you are suffering from an ailment.

Hydrotherapy

IN RECENT YEARS, water immersion has seen a twofold increase in popularity among expectant women, both as a means of gently exercising the body before birth and of easing discomfort and the pain of contractions during labour. Water therapy techniques can be used in the treatment of some common ailments.

> ### USES IN PREGNANCY
>
> * *Varicose veins*
> * *Skin problems*
> * *During labour*

HOW IT WORKS

Hydrotherapy, or exposure to water, in the form of natural springs, hot baths, steamrooms, saunas or ice massage, has been used to promote health and well-being from the very earliest civilizations. Water has a demonstrable ability to constrict or dilate blood vessels, depending on its temperature. Hot water raises body temperature, encouraging muscles to relax, soothing soreness and easing mental tension. Cold water stimulates blood circulation, reduces inflammation, and invigorates the skin. Hydrotherapy is often available at spas or health farms.

USES IN PREGNANCY

Exercise in water is particularly helpful during pregnancy, since extra weight you are carrying is offset by the buoyancy of the water, enabling muscles and joints to work with less strain. Many public swimming pools run exercise classes for pregnant women. Immersion in water in a birthing pool (*see page 103*), either rented privately for home or hospital use, or provided by the hospital, assists relaxation and relieves painful contractions.

TAKING CARE

Avoid steamrooms and hot baths in the first trimester and if you have raised blood pressure. In any case, limit sessions to ten minutes. A water birth must be supervised by a midwife or other qualified attendant.

BIRTHING POOL
Your midwife can monitor the baby while you are relaxing in a birthing pool.

Hypnotherapy

HYPNOSIS TODAY HAS THE RESPECT of conventional medicine and can help pregnant women to deal with common ailments and problems as well as fears about labour and birth.

HOW IT WORKS

Under hypnosis, the brain's conscious function is bypassed and the subconscious becomes extremely receptive to positive suggestion. Self-hypnosis can be taught by a hypnotherapist and is useful for relieving stress.

IN A TRANCE
During hypnosis a practitioner talks in a slow, soothing voice that encourages deep relaxation.

TREATMENT

The practitioner will ask about your health and your ability to cope with problems. Once the problem to be addressed has been identified, you will be put into a state of profound relaxation. You will thus be able to confront fears of the birth, learn pain management, overcome an addiction, or be relieved of symptoms.

Colour Therapy

COLOUR THERAPISTS claim that body cells, like colours themselves, oscillate at specific frequencies. Cells disturbed by illness or negative mental states may thus be "rebalanced" by exposure to specific hues.

COLOURS AND THEIR EFFECTS

- For fertility, energy, vitality
- For depression, low blood pressure
- For aches and pains
- To cleanse and purify
- For stress, raised blood pressure
- For spirituality and insight
- To treat addiction

TREATMENT

A colour therapist will study your medical history and colour preferences, but thereafter treatment may vary. Some therapists link colour with the *chakras* (*see page 142*), others interpret your "aura", while others perform "dowsing". You may be advised to wear certain colours or to visualize them, or you may be offered colour illumination therapy. This involves coloured light being directed at a particular part of the body or diffused all around you. A main colour is chosen, according to its effects on a particular organ, and may be used with its complementary colour. A course of colour therapy may last several weeks.

Osteopathy

BASED ON THE BELIEF that a healthy body depends on the proper functioning of the musculo-skeletal system, osteopathy uses manipulative techniques and massage to restore and maintain balance and the healthy function of bones and muscles. It may be of great benefit in relieving the aches and pains of pregnancy.

> ## USES IN PREGNANCY
>
> * *Backache & Symphysis pubic pain*
> * *Oedema & Carpal tunnel syndrome*

HOW IT WORKS

Misuse or trauma can upset the balance between muscles, joints, ligaments and nerves. An osteopath aims to restore and preserve optimal balance by easing muscle tension and restoring joint mobility. This balance is altered in pregnancy by changes in weight bearing, hormonal action and fluctuations in body fluid levels.

DIAGNOSIS & TREATMENT

An osteopath treats the whole person, not isolated conditions, investigating the reasons for imbalances in the musculo-skeletal system as well as the symptoms. Many pregnant women can obtain lasting relief for pain and other discomforts of pregnancy as well as for specific musculo-skeletal problems. After taking a full medical history and details of your lifestyle, work, and emotional health, an osteopath will observe

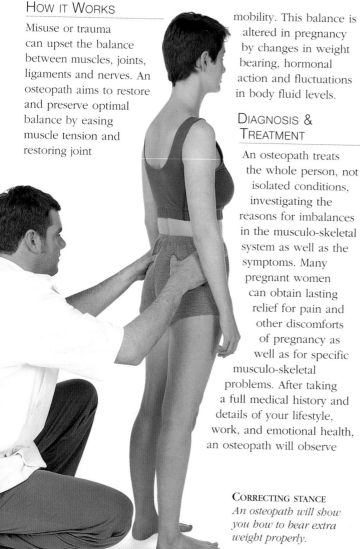

CORRECTING STANCE
An osteopath will show you how to bear extra weight properly.

your posture, weight distribution, and mobility. A diagnosis and treatment plan can then be established. This may include a final appointment six weeks after the birth of your baby. In the first trimester, osteopathy may be able to correct muscle shortening as a result of an increase in breast size and low back pain. In the second, it can help to correct a "pregnant posture" and referred hip or groin pain. Osteopathy may help to ease many ailments in the final trimester, including breathing difficulties, sciatica, restricted mobility, carpal tunnel syndrome and swollen ankles, indigestion and heartburn, symphysis pubic pain, and round ligament pain. After birth, osteopathy can treat back pain resulting from a poor delivery position, the trauma of delivery, or poor breastfeeding positions. Cranial osteopathy focuses on the part of the skull surrounding the brain and the fluid that protects membranes encasing the brain. It uses manipulative techniques similar to those of osteopathy and treats similar conditions.

Chiropractic

THE MOST WIDELY PRACTISED complementary therapy in the West, chiropractic maintains that any action of the spine affects all joints and muscles, and hence body systems. Manipulation is used to correct misalignment.

USES IN PREGNANCY

* *Backache, Symphysis pubic pain & Sciatica*

HOW IT WORKS

The spinal column is made up of 24 movable vertebrae, the sacrum and coccyx. Vertebral misalignment may interfere with nerves leaving the spinal column between joints, which causes pain. A chiropractor manipulates the spine, restoring full movement, relaxing the muscles and thus reducing inflammation. Harmony having been restored, the body's self-healing mechanisms will be able to function better.

TREATMENT

After taking details of your medical history, a practitioner will ask you to adopt various positions in order to evaluate spinal function. He or she may use a gentle thrust to free a joint, relieving the surrounding tissues. Back pain and nausea may be eased during pregnancy, and the pelvis and sacrum opened for birth. Realigning the spine releases uterine nerves so that they can function properly.

The Alexander Technique

TEACHING PEOPLE TO STAND, sit, and move in the way that nature intended is the goal of those instructing the Alexander technique. It may ease back pain and neck problems in pregnancy.

USES IN PREGNANCY

* *Respiratory problems*
* *Backache*

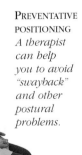

PREVENTATIVE POSITIONING
A therapist can help you to avoid "swayback" and other postural problems.

WHAT IT IS

This therapy was developed at the turn of the 19th century by an actor, Frederick Matthias Alexander. He had developed "patterns of misuse" in his shoulders and limbs, causing tension and impairing his vocal ability. He modified his posture by comparing it with that of a young child. The Alexander Technique is used during pregnancy in the treatment of pain caused by bad posture.

TREATMENT

An Alexander teacher begins by examining your stance and then repositions your body to achieve optimal posture, providing instruction as he or she does so. You learn a wide range of movements, including standing, sitting, lying, walking and lifting. Courses include 15–30 classes of 30–45 minutes each. Once it has been learnt, this technique can be applied anywhere and at any time.

Homeopathy

THE WORD HOMEOPATHY derives from the Greek *homoios* (like) and *pathos* (suffering). Based on the principle that "like cures like", homeopathy offers a healing method that is very popular among people seeking alternatives to conventional medicine.

HOW IT WORKS

Homeopathy is guided by the law of similars: "that which makes sick shall heal". In other words, a substance that produces the symptoms of a disease is also believed to cure it. Homeopathic remedies are derived from plants, minerals, animals and, more rarely, the disease itself. First, a substance is soaked in alcohol to extract the active ingredients. The resulting "mother tincture" is diluted tens or hundreds of times, and succussed, or shaken vigorously, to "potentize" the mixture and increase its healing powers. The number of a remedy indicates how many times it has been diluted and succussed. Paradoxically, the more a remedy is diluted, the greater its potency. The remedy is used to coat a small, tasteless pill which dissolves on the tongue.

DIAGNOSIS & TREATMENT

Homeopaths view symptoms of illness as signs that the body is using its powers of self-healing to fight a disease. The symptoms are regarded as a reliable guide to the remedy needed to activate this self-healing power. Each remedy is specific to a particular patient at a particular time. Ailments are thought to result from an imbalance in the body's integrative "vital force". A classical homeopath will assess all the factors that constitute your makeup – physical, intellectual and emotional. Your first appointment may therefore last up to two hours. The practitioner will record details of your physical traits, temperament and habits, likes, dislikes and

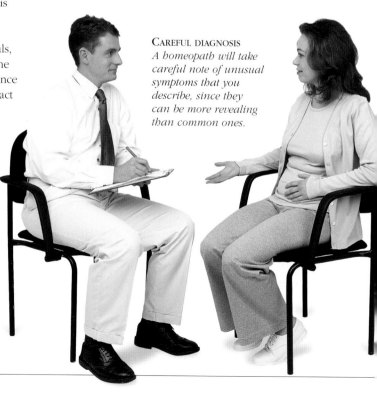

CAREFUL DIAGNOSIS
A homeopath will take careful note of unusual symptoms that you describe, since they can be more revealing than common ones.

POPULAR HOMEOPATHIC REMEDIES

	CONDITION	SELF-HELP REMEDY
1ST TRIMESTER	Morning sickness	*Ipecac., Nux vomica, Pulsatilla; see page 37*
	Tiredness	*Calc. carb., Arsen. alb., Nux vomica*
	Threat of miscarriage	*Ipecac., Kali carb., Pulsatilla; see page 43*
2ND & 3RD TRIMESTERS	Heartburn	*Carbo veg., Nux vomica, Pulsatilla; see page 55*
	Headaches	*Aconite, Belladonna, Bryonia; see page 61*
	Constipation	*Bryonia, Nux vomica, Sepia, Sulphur*
	Haemorrhoids	*Nux vomica, Hamamelis, Sepia; see page 63*
	Sleeplessness	*Gelsemium*
	Skin complaints	*Sulphur, Graphites*
LABOUR	Emotional state	*Pulsatilla; see page 109*
	Pain	*Caulophyllum, page 97; Pulsatilla, Chamomilla, page 103*
POSTNATAL	Breastfeeding problems	*Belladonna, Pulsatilla, Bryonia; see page 123*
	Bruising	*Arnica; see page 125*
	Caesarean section	*Arnica, Opium; see page 127*

fears as well as your medical history and current symptoms. How these symptoms are affected by time of day, atmospheric conditions, taking food and drink, rest and many other factors is significant. Some questions may seem unusual or irrelevant, but they are necessary for a practitioner to be able to build up a picture of your unique characteristics. This permits assessment of your "consitutional type", which, along with your symptoms, is used to determine which of the 2,000 remedies in the homeopathic repertory will be the most suitable. A remedy may be constitutional – for a chronic, underlying condition, or acute – for the immediate symptoms of an ailment. A few

consultations may be necessary, depending on your recovery, and the prescription may be changed at a subsequent visit. A remedy is usually taken in tablet form between meals. No food or drink should be consumed for at least 10–15 minutes afterwards. An exercise programme, dietary measures, and lifestyle changes may also be recommended. Symptoms may worsen slightly before they improve. If there is a sustained improvement, you should stop taking the remedy.

HOMEOPATHIC SELF-HELP

There are many homeopathic remedies available over the counter and self-help books to guide you in self-diagnosis. When you are self-prescribing,

list your symptoms and their characteristics before choosing a remedy. If taking over-the-counter remedies, follow the manufacturers' instructions about dosage and usage.

CAUTIONS

If your pregnancy is normal and healthy, self-help remedies are safe. Consult your midwife, doctor or a homeopath if you are unsure about using them. Certain substances, such as coffee, eucalyptus, menthol, spearmint and peppermint (including many proprietary toothpastes and mouthwashes) may neutralize remedies and should be avoided.

Western Herbalism

HERBS HAVE BEEN USED for thousands of years to ease labour pain and speed recovery from childbirth. Herbal lore was practised and passed down by wise women and midwives. As science advanced in Europe, herbalism declined, but has recently re-emerged.

USES IN PREGNANCY

* *Morning sickness*
* *Constipation*
* *Stress & Anxiety*
* *Sleeplessness*
* *Skin problems*
* *Breastfeeding problems*

HOW IT WORKS

Many modern pharmaceutical products are derived from herbal remedies. Whereas synthesized drugs are based on isolated plant extracts, herbal remedies derive from whole parts of a plant, such as leaves or roots. Herbalists claim that a plant's many chemical ingredients work in synergy, producing therapeutic effects that are greater when those ingredients are used together rather than separately. A herbal remedy is both gentler than a conventional drug and more effective in meeting the body's needs as a whole. A remedy will be tailored to the needs of an individual rather than just their list of symptoms.

DIAGNOSIS & TREATMENT

A first visit to a herbalist usually lasts for an hour. The practitioner will study your medical history in great detail as well as carrying out a physical examination, paying particular attention to body systems such as respiration, digestion and circulation. If appropriate, one or more remedies may be prescribed. The herbalist may make up the remedies or they may be bought from a reputable supplier. The practitioner may advise you on diet, exercise and aspects of lifestyle as well, and may recommend a follow-up visit. Herbal remedies may take longer to be effective than conventional drugs, and need to be taken for a week or two after symptoms have gone.

HERBAL SELF-HELP

Plant remedies should be used under the supervision of a professional medical herbalist (*see* Caution, *opposite*). If you are taking conventional drugs,

MAKING A HERBAL INFUSION

Suitable containers include a teapot, cup or vacuum flask (avoid using aluminium, tin or plastic containers). Plant parts that are suitable for infusion are leaves, flowers or seeds, depending on the particular remedy. For maximum benefit, be sure to obtain the freshest material possible, even if that material is dried. Fill the container with boiling water. Place 5 g (1 tsp) of the dried plant material in the pot and add 1 cup of boiling water. Replace the lid and leave for 10–15 minutes. Let it cool, strain it and drink. To make a larger quantity, use about 30 g (1$1/4$ oz) of the dried plant to 500 ml (18 fl oz) water.

Popular Herbal Remedies

	Condition	Self-Help Remedy
1ST TRIMESTER	Morning sickness	*Chamomile, fennel, ginger, peppermint; see page 37*
	Threat of miscarriage	*Ginger; see page 43*
	Swollen joints	*Cabbage, dandelion, nettle; see page 87*
	Anaemia	*Nettle; see page 57*
2ND & 3RD TRIMESTERS	Constipation	*Dandelion; see page 63*
	Haemorrhoids	*St John's wort; see page 63*
	Headaches	*Chamomile, ginger; see page 61*
	Heartburn	*Fennel, chamomile, peppermint; see page 55*
LABOUR	Preparation	*Raspberry leaf; see pages 96–7*
	Relaxation; pain relief	*Chamomile*
POSTNATAL	Care of the perineum	*Calendula, witch hazel; see page 125*
	Postnatal depression	*Rosemary, vervain, borage, St John's wort; see page129*
	Breast engorgement	*Cabbage; see page 123*
	Lactation	*Fennel; see page 97*

nform your doctor that you are considering herbal treatment, nd likewise let your herbalist know about any conventional medication. A small number of herbs are so gentle that, taken n moderation, they may be used for the self-treatment of many common ailments. These nclude lime blossom, fennel, hamomile, lemon balm, red lover, rosehip, peppermint, porage and ginger. However, always make sure that you ollow the manufacturer's nstructions carefully when using over-the-counter remedies.

Using Herbal Treatments

Herbal self-treatments in the orm of infusions (*see opposite*), decoctions, creams, ointments, poultices, compresses, powders and capsules may help to ease many common complaints of pregnancy. Herbs such as lavender, lime flower, orange flower and rose petals can simply be tied in muslin bags and held under running water to make a fragrant, soothing bath to relieve stress, for example. A compress, often used to heal wounds, is made by dissolving the appropriate herb extract in hot water, soaking a soft cotton pad or cloth and placing it on the affected area. A poultice is similar but the whole herb is applied, not just an extract. Compresses and poultices are usually hot but may be cold. Several herbs are available as ointments and creams for direct application. Calendula ointment is good for cracked, sore nipples, for example. Some plants can be used as they are: grated raw potato on a haemorrhoid, for example, or cabbage leaves to relieve engorged breasts.

Caution

There are many herbs that should not be used at all during pregnancy because of their potentially adverse effects on the developing foetus. Others should only be used under the guidance of a professional medical herbalist. If you are in doubt about taking any plant remedies during pregnancy, consult your doctor, midwife or a qualified herbalist.

Aromatherapy

THE TERM "AROMATHERAPY" was coined in the 1920s by Réné-Maurice Gattefossé, a French chemist who extensively investigated the healing properties of plant oils. Today the therapy combines this knowledge with the tradition of healing massage.

USES IN PREGNANCY

* *Hyperemesis*
* *Headaches*
* *Sleeplessness*
* *Raised blood pressure*
* *During labour*
* *Perineal care*

HOW IT WORKS

Gattefossé began his work after accidentally burning his hand. Having applied oil of lavender to the wound, he found that the skin healed rapidly with no scarring. Obtained primarily by steam distillation from aromatic plants, herbs and spices, essential oils contain a variety of volatile organic compounds. When inhaled, it is believed, these substances pass into the bloodstream and then into the nervous system, where they act upon the brain's limbic system. This is linked to instinctive behaviour, the emotions and the control of hormones. Different oils have different effects: some are calming, others stimulating. Therapists maintain that the constituents of essential oils have therapeutic properties that bring benefits to health.

DIAGNOSIS & TREATMENT

Ensure that an aromatherapist is fully qualified. At your first session, the practitioner will study your medical history and lifestyle. Oils will be selected for their specific effects. It is important, however, that the aromas are pleasing to the patient. A key aspect of the skill of aromatherapy is in the blending. Up to five oils may be combined, the total effect being greater than that of each oil used separately. Essential oils are always diluted in a carrier oil before being applied to the skin. Common carrier oils include almond, sunflower and grapeseed. Professional treatment usually takes the form of therapeutic massage based on Swedish massage techniques. For self-treatment, diluted oils may be added to a bath, steam inhalations or compresses.

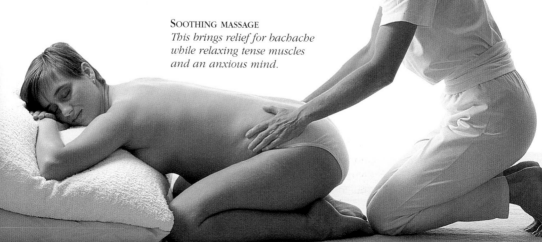

SOOTHING MASSAGE
This brings relief for backache while relaxing tense muscles and an anxious mind.

POPULAR ESSENTIAL OILS

	CONDITION	SELF-HELP REMEDY
1ST, 2ND & 3RD TRIMESTERS	Hyperemesis	*Bergamot, citrus oils; see page 39*
	Heartburn	*Lavender, chamomile; see page 55*
	Headaches	*Lavender; see page 61*
	Constipation	*Mandarin, orange; see page 63*
	Thrush	*Tea tree, chamomile; see page 64*
	Sleeplessness	*Mandarin, lavender; see page 79*
	Anxiety	*Chamomile, sandalwood; see page 83*
	Raised blood pressure	*Chamomile, lavender;* see page 85
LABOUR	Pain relief	*Lavender, chamomile, eucalyptus; see page 103*
	Slow labour	*Clary sage; see page 103*
POSTNATAL	Perineal care	*Lavender, cypress; see page 125*
	Postnatal depression	*Jasmine, lemon, lime, grapefruit; see page 129*
	Engorgement	*Fennel, lavender, rose; see page 123*
	Stretch marks	*Mandarin; see page 81*

An oil may also be heated in a burner to release the vapours into the atmosphere.

OILS IN PREGNANCY

While many essential oils are of benefit during pregnancy, in labour and after the birth for the treatment of a range of ailments from digestive problems to stress-related disorders, it is important to take precautions. There is great debate about which oils should or should not be used in pregnancy. Some people believe that it is inadvisable to use them in the first trimester, but many oils are safe for treating common ailments (*see* Caution, *right*). Aromatherapy obviously has great self-help potential, used

sensibly. Never take oils by mouth; use pure organic oils; follow instructions carefully; and do not be tempted to use unknown oils. Consult your midwife or doctor before using essential oils. A low dilution of oil is often recommended for use during pregnancy; that is five drops essential oil to 20 ml (4 tsp) carrier oil. Most oils will sting if they get into the eyes. If this happens, flush them out with warm water. Oils tend to persist on fingers for a long time and may irritate sensitive skin, especially if they are black peppermint, camphor, clove, eucalyptus, ginger, juniper, pimento, sage, spearmint or thyme. Due to the potential for irritation of a newborn's eyes,

oils must not be used in a birthing pool. Do not use essential oils, even if diluted, on a newborn baby's skin.

CAUTION

Some oils are perfectly safe to use throughout pregnancy, including ginger, neroli, petit grain, rosewood, sandalwood, tea tree, and ylang ylang. Some should be used with slight caution: bergamot, chamomile, cypress, frankincense, geranium, lavender, marjoram and peppermint. Others need great caution, such as clary sage and rosemary; only use just before or during labour.

Flower Remedies

THE USE OF FLOWER REMEDIES was first recorded in ancient Egypt. Traditionally self-prescribed, and most often for emotional problems, flower essences have become increasingly popular in recent years, even though their effectiveness is unproven.

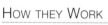

USES IN PREGNANCY

* Hyperemesis
* Threatened miscarriage
* Sleeplessness
* Depression
* Stress & Anxiety
* Postnatal depression

HOW THEY WORK

In the 1930s, physician and homeopath Edward Bach revived the ancient therapeutic use of flower essences. Today, essences are derived from native plants the world over – from Alaska to the Australian bush. Bach's own distillations, made by infusing plant parts in spring water and preserving their essence in alcohol, are prescribed for an individual rather than for a disease, in the belief that a person's emotional and spiritual state and their personality are responsible for health and well-being.

TREATMENT

There are 38 Bach remedies. Each one consists of a single essence intended for a particular mood, emotional state or aspect of the personality, except for the Rescue Remedy blend, which is recommended for mental shock or panic. Up to six or seven remedies may be combined, depending on specific needs.

Since remedies are preserved in brandy, it is important during pregnancy to follow dosage instructions carefully. Put two drops of each remedy selected into a 30 ml (1 fl oz) bottle and top up with mineral water or fruit juice. Take four drops at least four times daily until your condition improves. For a passing mood, add two to four drops to a glass of water and sip at intervals during the day.

CHOOSING REMEDIES

Descriptions of remedies tend to reflect their indications, so moods are often described negatively. Remedy choice is based on a person's assessment of emotional state, mood and personality. In the first two trimesters, remedies include: mimulus, for fear of pain and something going wrong; walnut, for adjustment to change; and olive, for exhaustion. In the third trimester, rock rose is for terrifying thoughts; while

TAKING FLOWER REMEDIES
Remedies can be diluted in fruit juice or mineral water, or dripped directly on to the tongue.

in labour, Rescue Remedy is for calming the mind and easing pain and shock. Postnatally, star of Bethlehem is for the shock of a traumatic birth; mustard, gentian and sweet chestnut are for depression; clematis is for detachment from reality; and elm is for feelings of overwhelming responsibility.

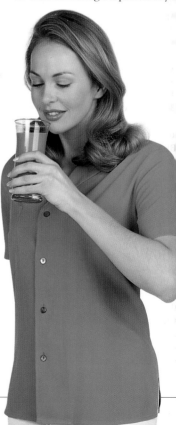

Glossary

Acupoint in Traditional Chinese Medicine, a point on a meridian at which the flow of *qi* is accessed by, for example, applying pressure or an acupuncture needle.

Acute describing the symptoms of an ailment that come on suddenly and change quickly.

Adrenaline a hormone that is released by the body in response to exercise, stress and emotions such as fear or panic.

Aerobic describing exercise intended to increase the amount of oxygen used by the body.

Alveoli small air sacs in the lungs where gases are exhanged bewteen the lungs and the blood.

Antacid a drug that helps to neutralize the acid secreted in the stomach.

Anti-oxidant a substance that inhibits the action of free radicals, which can damage genetic material and adversely affect cholesterol.

Apgar score a system devised to assess the physical well-being of a newborn baby. Heart rate, breathing, skin colour, muscle tone and action to stimule are assessed at one minute and five minutes after the birth.

Beta carotene a nutrient found in yellow- and orange-coloured fruits and vegetables.

Blood sugar glucose carried to all tissues by the blood and the main source of energy for the body.

Braxton Hicks contractions short, painless contractions of the uterus that occur throughout pregnancy and do not affect the cervix.

Chakras in yoga, spiritual centre of energy in the body.

Cholesterol a substance involved in the trasportation of fat in the bloodstream.

Chronic describing symptoms of an ailment that last a long time and change slowly.

Colostrum the fluid produced by the breasts after the birth of a baby prior to milk production.

Compress a soft cloth pad soaked in a hot herbal extract and applied to a wound or painful area.

Constitutional treatment in homeopathy, the prescription of a remedy based on an assessment of a person's physical, intellectual and emotional make-up as well as their chronic ailments.

Decoction a plant extract obtained by simmering parts of the plant for up to one hour.

Diuretic describing something that stimulates urine production.

Douche the direction of water on to the body or into a body cavity for cleansing or healing purposes.

Endorphins substances, similar to morphine, produced by the body to relieve pain.

Episiotomy a surgical incision made during labout to make the delivery of the baby easier.

Fatty acids basic constituents of fats and oils. Not all are made by the body and need to be provided by the diet.

Folate a B vitamin.

Folic acid the synthetic form of folate.

Hyperemesis excessive vomiting.

Hypertension abnormally high blood pressure.

Infusion a plant extract obtained by adding freshly boiled water to the leaves and flowers of the plant and straining after ten minutes.

Meconium the thick, greenish-black faeces passed by a baby in the first few days after the birth.

Meridian in Traditional Chinese Medicine, a channel running through the body that transpots *qi*.

Neurotransmitter a chemical substance released by a nerve fibre that permits the transferance of impulses to muscles or other nerves.

Obstetric cholestasis severe itching of the skin requiring conventional medical attention.

Oedema swelling of the hands, feet, face and other areas due to the abnormal accumulation of fluid in body tissues.

Oxytocin a hormone produced during labout to stimulate the production of milk in the breasts.

Perineum the areas between the thighs that lies behind the vagina and in front of the anus. diam nonummy nibh euismod

Placenta previa the location of the placenta close to or overlapping the cervix, reducing the likelihood of vaginal delivery.

Poultice the application of a plant, usually hot by being boiled for a few minutes, directly to a wound or painful area.

Qi in Traditional Chinese Medicine, the life energy that flows through the body.

Rhinitus inflammation of mucous membranes of the nose due to allergy, for example hayfever.

Sacroiliac relating to the functioning of the sacrum and ilium bones in the pelvis.

Surfactant a wetting agent that reduces surface tension, for example in the linings of the alveoli in the lungs.

Saturated fat fat that contains fatty acids and cholesterol.

Thrombosis the formation of a clot in a blood vessel.

Tincture a plant extract obtained by steeping parts of a plant in a mixture of alcohol and water.

Tissue salts vital minerals, obtained and prescribed in a similar way to homeopathic remedies.

Toxins waste products produced by the body and environmental poisons.

Transcendental meditation a method of meditation that induces relaxed state of consciousness and spiritual well-being by the repetition of a mantra.

Trimester a three-month period.

Unsaturated fat a fat that contains fatty acids but no cholesterol.

Vernix a white, greasy substance covering a newborn baby.

156

Index

Useful Contacts

National Childbirth Trust (NCT)
Alexandra House, Oldham Terrace
London W3 6NH
020 8992 8637

Eating for Pregnancy Helpline
0114 2424084

Drinkline: the National Alcohol
Helpline
0345 320202

Quitline (smoking)
020 7487 3000 (England)
011222 641888 (Wales)
0800 848484 (Scotland)
01232 663281 (N. Ireland)

The Miscarriage Association
c/o Clayton Hospital
Northgate, Wakefield
North Yorkshire WF1 3JS

Twins & Multiple Birth Association
PO Box 30
Little Sutton
South Wirral L66 1TH
Advice line: 01732 868000

Association of Breastfeeding Mothers
PO Box 441
St Albans
Herts AL4 0AS

Caesarean Support Network
55 Cooil Drive
Douglas, Isle of Man
01624 661269 (after 6 pm)

Association for Postnatal Illness
25 Jerden Place
London SW6 1BE
020 7386 0868

Stillbirth & Neonatal Death Society
(SANDS)
28 Portland Place
London W1N 4DE

Association of Spina Bifida and
Hydrocephalus Helpline
01733 555988

Down's Syndrome Association
155 Mitcham Road
London SW17 9PG

Institute for Complementary
Medicine
PO Box 194
London SE16 1QZ

British Acupuncture Council
Park House
206–208 Latimer Road
London W10 6RE

The Shiatsu Society
Interchange Studios, Dalby Street
London NW5 3NQ

British Reflexology Association
Monks Orchard, Whitbourne
Worcester WR6 5RB

British Wheel of Yoga
Central Office

1 Hamilton Place
Boston Road, Sleaford
Lincolnshire NG34 7ES

British Hypnotherapy Association
1 Wythburn Place
London W1H 5WL

General Council and Register of
Osteopaths
56 London Street
Reading
Berkshire RG1 4SQ

British Chiropractic Association
Equity House, 29 Whitley Street
Reading
Berkshire RG2 0EG

Society of Teachers of the Alexander
Technique
20 London House, 266 Fulham Road
London SQ10 9EL

British Homeopathic Association
27a Devonshire Street
London W1N 1RJ
020 7935 2163

National Institute of Medical
Herbalists
56 Longbrook Street
Exeter
Devon EX4 6AH

Zita West Pregnancy Products
0870 1668899

Acknowledgments

The author would like to thank the following people for their help and support during the production of this book: her family – Robert, Sofie and Jack; Sharon Bayliss; Jude Garlick, Dawn Terrey, Andy Crawford and all the mothers who were photographed; Martin Watt, medical herbalist and essential oil educator; Sylvia Baddeley (exercise consultant); Denise Tiran (aromatherapy); Ian Spiers (reiki); Esther Wai Lin (Shiatsu); Charmaine Culling (osteopathy); Judy Howard (flower remedies); Hazel Pelham and Iain Cloughley (nutrition) and Barbara Geraghty (homeopathy).

Dorling Kindersley would like to thank Sue Bosanko, Monica Chakraverty and Christa Weil for their editorial assistance; and Jayne Jones, Rachana Shah, Elaine Monaghan, Anne Renel and David Ball for their design assistance.

Models
Nicola August, Rimi Hozumi and partner, Karen McCracken, Germaine Morgan, Megan Murphy-Patel, Tracey Ward and partner, Nasim Mawji, Jane Jones and Rachana Shah.